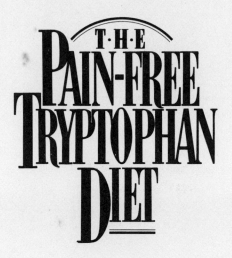

ROBERT L. POLLACK, PH.D.
WITH GERRY HUNT & MARCIA ROSEN

T·H·E
PAIN-FREE
TRYPTOPHAN
DIET

Foreword by
ALAN P. BERG, Ph.D., M.D.

WARNER BOOKS

A Warner Communications Company

Warner Books, Inc., 666 Fifth Avenue, New York, NY 10103

w A Warner Communications Company

Printed in the United States of America
First Printing: May 1986
10 9 8 7 6 5 4 3 2 1

Designed by Giorgetta Bell McRee

Library of Congress Cataloging-in-Publication Data

Pollack, Robert L.
  The pain-free tryptophan diet.

  1. Pain—Diet therapy—Popular works. 2. High-
tryptophan diet. 3. Reducing diets. I. Hunt, Gerry.
II. Rosen, Marcia. III. Title. [DNLM: 1. Diet—
popular works. 2. Pain—diet therapy—popular works.
3. Tryptophan—therapeutic use—popular works.
QU 60 P771p]
RB127.P65 1986   616′.0472   85-43176
ISBN 0-446-51317-2

ACKNOWLEDGMENTS

The authors would like to acknowledge the ground-breaking studies of Dr. Richard J. Wurtman, M.D., director of the Laboratory of Neuroendocrine Regulation, and his wife and coscientist, Dr. Judith J. Wurtman, Ph.D., both of MIT, Cambridge, Massachusetts. Without their pioneering breakthroughs, much of the state-of-the-art understanding of the tryptophan-nutrition connection would not exist today.

The inspiration for this manuscript would not have been possible without the consultation, help, and advice of Dr. Samuel Seltzer of the Maxillofacial Pain Control Center at Temple University, whose original, illuminating studies into tryptophan and pain opened the Pain-Free Diet door.

We would like to thank Kathleen Malley, our editor at Warner Books, for her insight into recognizing the potential of the Pain-Free Diet and her perseverance in the publishing process; and also our agents Adele Leone and Richard Monaco, of New York City, for their professionalism, enthusiasm, and most of all their support.

v

CONTENTS

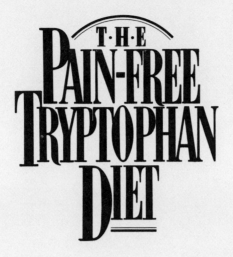

T·H·E
PAIN-FREE
TRYPTOPHAN
DIET

FOREWORD

As both a research chemist and a practicing physician, I was initially skeptical that something as commonplace as food could relieve or prevent pain. After all, people with chronic pain seem to eat no differently than other people. Such an imposing target for such an apparently small weapon! Nevertheless, my curiosity was aroused. Far from being new or radical, the experimental support for such an idea had been accumulating steadily since the 1950s and now rests on a solid and logical foundation.

The key is tryptophan, a common ingredient of proteins from both plant and animal sources, and a small but crucial part of the human diet for over two million years as a species. As Dr. Pollack elaborates, we now know why tryptophan reduces pain and how to design our diets to achieve the optimal tryptophan intake. The approach is simple yet profound. It works. Remarkably, while reducing pain the Pain-Free Diet not only helps to normalize weight but in doing so protects the heart as well. It can also relieve some people's depression and promote good sleep.

1

Pain is so common that we have developed many names for it, reflecting its various locations, causes, and sensations: an apparent perplexity of discomforting feelings. Over the centuries many cultures have tried to get rid of pain. There are chants, relaxation therapy, hypnosis and acupuncture, drugs as different as aspirin and heroin, and even neurosurgery. The power of diet is that it can alter those brain chemicals which modulate our perception of pain. The wrong diet can make any kind of pain worse; the Pain-Free Diet can make any kind of pain less and therefore should be considered a key factor in any pain-control program.

It is clear that numerous people stand to benefit. For some, the Pain-Free Diet will become their first line of defense against chronic pain. For many others, using the diet will allow a reduction in the use of pain medications or other therapies. For some, it may permit, perhaps for the first time, the safe and effective elimination of daily pain medications. Unfortunately, a few may not benefit to the same extent, and for these people alternate therapies will have to play a major role in their lives.

A natural question is: Will the Pain-Free Diet help reduce my kind of pain? The encouraging answer is a clear yes for almost all kinds of pain. Dr. Pollack's own studies at prestigious Temple University in Philadelphia showed improvement in pain as diverse as atypical facial neuralgia, temporomandibular joint (TMJ) pain-dysfunction syndrome, and cervical osteoarthritis. Many patients had almost given up hope of ever finding relief. Other investigators have shown that tryptophan reduces pain in settings as diverse as migraine headaches, the pain of deep-seated arthritis, the pain following surgery, and the ischemic pain that sometimes plagues those with poor circulation.

The other necessary natural question is: How safe is it? Physicians everywhere are admonished, first and foremost, to do no harm. The Pain-Free Diet meets this stringent test. It is superbly safe. Even in quite large doses, tryptophan has no significant toxic effects. There is even good reason to believe that a true excess is impossible since the body simply disposes of any amounts over and above its needs.

Despite its proven safety, Dr. Pollack still suggests the Pain-Free Diet be used with the concurrence of the family physician. This makes sense to me for several reasons. Some may find the physician's validation of the diet's safety reassuring to them. Some may want help in determining their optimum calorie level. Others may be taking one or more medications the effectiveness of which is enhanced as a result of the diet, such that, after a while, less drugs should be taken. This may be particularly important for those taking insulin, tricyclic antidepressants, mono-amine-oxidase inhibitors, and perhaps some antihypertensive medications. Last, we are coming to realize just how unique each of us is in regard to our nutritional needs. In this spirit our family doctor can help "fine tune" our diet.

Dr. Pollack has helped pioneer a safe and sane nutritional approach to the control of pain. As set forth here, you will learn why the proper balance of protein, carbohydrate, and fat reduces pain; you will also learn how to design your own diet based on these principles, and how to do so with dietary interest and variety.

There is more, but read on and find out for yourself.

—Alan P. Berg, Ph.D., M.D.

INTRODUCTION

PAIN: YOU ARE NOT ALONE

Pain is the silent assailant; it can strike at any time, any place. It's unpredictable and it can completely incapacitate a person for seconds, minutes, hours, or even years. For many sufferers, pain is an unfortunate daily fact of life, a cross they expect to bear for a lifetime.

Pain comes in many forms. It can range from a split-second excruciating attack, or a searing hurt that may last for hours, to a dull but grindingly agonizing throb that's with you all the time. Words we commonly use to describe the type of pain we feel include *pinching*, *pulsing*, *rasping*, *grating*, *gnawing*, *throbbing*, *burning*, and *wrenching*. The one thing that all pain has in common is that you know it is there.

But new research breakthroughs in the nutrition and biochemical fields show you have built-in capacities to cope with pain; you can learn how to reduce it, and many pain

5

sufferers can suddenly find themselves without pain for the first time in years.

The Pain-Free Diet is the ultimate pain-reduction and weight-control plan. It is the only diet developed to harness nature's nutritional ability to control pain. And unlike other diets, it incorporates four different nutritional programs to suit your desired weight goals: not just a safe and sure remedy for weight control, but a new scientific approach to boosting the body's own remarkable pain-defense systems through correct nutrition.

If the solution is as simple as what you eat and how you eat, how is it that nobody has developed a plan like this before? It's only in the past few years that biochemists and researchers in the nutritional field have recognized the importance of one of our essential amino acids and its critical role in the control of pain.

The amino acid is tryptophan (pronounced trip-toe-fan), a nutrient that we derive from protein in many foods, and one we can also take in dietary supplement form. Tryptophan is the key to our pain threshold—the amount of pain we can comfortably endure. The Pain-Free Diet is designed to increase tryptophan levels in the body safely with a correct balance of enjoyable foods in a diet that promotes its optimum utilization.

Research has shown how tryptophan-boosting, working hand in hand with a nutritionally balanced diet plan to permit its maximum efficiency, can reduce pain and increase our tolerance to it. But more about the biochemical wonders of tryptophan later.

THE PAIN PICTURE

There are over 100 million people in the United States suffering from pain this very day, ranging from headaches and migraine to backaches, muscular problems, angina, coronary disease, and cancer. It's a massive problem not only for the pain sufferers but for their families and the physicians and other health care professionals who have to cope with it.

Back pain alone—America's number-one chronic-pain problem—accounts for more than eighteen million visits to physicians' offices each year. And migraine and other headaches occupy more than twelve million hours of doctors' time.

Coated, capsuled, buffered over-the-counter (otc) pain-relief preparations, with their varying pain-reducing ingredients and differing price tags, may promise hours of relief, but when the chips are down none of these preparations is more effective per gram than our old faithful aspirin.

However, with aspirin there is, unfortunately for some people, the problem of adverse reactions, especially in the gastrointestinal system. Aspirin can cause internal bleeding in the stomach and gastrointestinal discomfort.

But with thirty-six million arthritis sufferers in the United States, seventy million people with agonizing back pain, and about twenty-four million who suffer from blinding migraines and headaches, it's hardly suprising that there is such an overwhelming demand for over-the-counter medications.

There are stronger prescription drugs, of course, but many of these also have unwanted side effects. They can be extremely expensive, especially if they are prescribed over the long term. Another time-related problem is that the body can adjust to many drugs and their initial effectiveness is reduced with use, often meaning that repeatedly higher doses of the drug then have to be administered.

Medications may be perfectly sound remedies for temporary relief, but they miss the point: They do not go to the root of the problem. Taking painkillers is like using an air freshener to disguise the source of a bad odor.

It's estimated that pain victims spend a whopping $900 million a year in the United States for analgesic pills, powders, potions, and soothing salves, and then there's an additional $70 billion in medical costs, lost workdays, and compensation. Are those staggering financial figures really necessary?

One of the most promising modern scientific approaches to pain relief is to attack the problem from within . . . utilizing nutrition. In fact, a recent report to the White House stressed that the most promising avenues for future pain management would be through nutrition.

This is exactly what the Pain-Free Diet is all about. Utilizing nutrition and the natural biomedical benefits of tryptophan, you can learn to harness your body's natural pain-free potential.

FOOD PAIN

The overall story of pain is extremely complex, and the one single item that makes it even more so is food! Many pain patients suffer intermittent and even daily pain that stems directly from some of the foods they regularly eat. Surprised? So are many physicians who have been unaware of the source of this pain problem.

It's also little wonder many people—including their health care professionals—have problems pinpointing the source of certain pains. This is because food-triggered pain has until recently been very much ignored.

We call these edible adversaries "foods that eat you." They are very real, and for many people very potent pain sources. Their effects can result in chronic headaches, debilitating migraines, and severe muscular discomfort—and they're literally everywhere in our daily diets, from chocolate to shellfish, coffee to champagne. The Pain-Free Diet will show you how to recognize and eliminate these dietary causes of pain.

WEIGHT PAIN

Weight is also another important factor in the intensity of pain. It doesn't take a Rhodes Scholar to recognize that if a 200-pound man with chronic lower lumbar pain is carrying 35 pounds of excess flab on his body he's courting trouble. It's pretty much as if he were walking around all day with a 25-pound sack of potatoes slung across his shoulders. Remember how heavy 25 pounds feels when you try to lift it! Obviously, this can do nothing but inflame an already painful problem and escalate it into one that may become totally debilitating. Bad backs and hips are particularly vulnerable to excess weight.

That same overweight pain victim is probably missing valuable workdays because of his problem. In total we lose 700 million workdays a year through pain, and much of this can be avoided with sensible nutrition. A well-balanced nutritional diet, producing and maintaing an ideal weight, is another vital benefit of the Pain-Free Diet.

EXERCISE AND PAIN

Exercise is also a powerful weapon in our arsenal against pain. No, it doesn't have to be the strenuous pull, push, and tug variety, which for many pain sufferers may not only be excruciatingly unbearable but impossible. Exercise that combats pain can be as simple as special breathing exercises and armchair calisthenics.

An exercise approach to pain management can have a dual beneficial effect. Physical motion that keeps your muscles and joints limber and flexible is more valuable than that which builds unnecessary strength. The National Arthritis Foundation suggests some wonderfully easy pain-free exercises, and these will be found in our toning-up section in Chapter 12.

In addition, exercise has the ability to reduce pain by promoting endorphin release by the brain—sending a surge of natural "analgesics" into the bloodstream.

CHRONIC PAIN

Who is the average chronic-pain victim? Estimates show this person to have suffered for seven years, undergone from three to five major operations, and spent between $50,000 to $100,000 in medical bills. This person has also taken countless drugs, including muscle relaxants, tranquilizers, and potent narcotics, in the quest to banish pain.

Another sorry statistic is that this individual also stands a fifty-fifty chance of acquiring a drug-dependent habit along the way. And, remember, this is the *average* chronic-pain sufferer.

There are six major categories into which chronic pain falls.

1. *Muscle and joint pain.* This includes our well-known low back pain and accounts for the largest number of pain sufferers. Arthritis, bursitis, and tendonitis are also muscle- and joint-pain problems.

2. *Vascular pain.* This includes migraines and headaches that arise from the dilation, and sometimes constriction, of the major blood vessels around the brain. The brain itself can be punched, pummeled, twisted, squeezed, and even pierced without your ever feeling

pain—but the surrounding structures and vessels are highly sensitive to pain. Atherosclerotic deposits that build up in the vascular system can also cause agonizing pain.

3. *Neuralgia.* This pain stems from problems arising in the peripheral nerves. One of the most excruciating pain problems, trigeminal neuralgia, or tic douloureux, which can affect either side of the face, is a neuralgia. Its punishment is so intensely painful that trigeminal neuralgia is believed to be *the* leading cause of pain-related suicides.

4. *Causalgia.* This is a searing pain that accompanies or appears after a sudden shock to the peripheral nervous system. Typical examples would be a bullet wound or traumatic injuries produced during the violence of a serious automobile accident. The pain, often described as feeling similar to having boiling water or lighted cigarettes applied to the affected area, may take as long as six months or a year to disappear, but in 25 percent of cases the pain residue from the initial wound can last much longer.

5. *Phantom limb pain.* This bizarre syndrome is still not fully understood, but it appears sometimes when a limb has been amputated. The victim feels all the agonizing pain as if the limb were still present and undergoing injury. Even people paralyzed by spinal cord injuries—who should not be feeling pain at all because of severed nerves—can experience what is termed paraplegic pain. This chronic pain may develop into forms of cramping, burning, or shooting pain.

6. *Terminal-cancer pain.* Major organs can be blocked and "strangled" by the rapidly growing cancers, and surrounding tissue destruction results in pain. Cancers

often spread to the spine, where they destroy bone and compress nerves, causing additional intense pain.

PERCEPTION OF PAIN

A new understanding of pain shows that the severity of pain can differ depending on the way we perceive it. In other words, a little bit of mind over matter can often relieve the pain or make it less important, allowing us a greater ability to ignore it.

A curious phenomenon noticed repeatedly during the two great wars was the ability of the wounded battlefield soldier to tolerate pain. Field physicians were constantly amazed at the soldiers' ability to ignore the pain of mangled limbs and internal injuries.

Obviously, the field surgeons concluded, something was going on that either masked the pain or made it more bearable. One theory held that the relief that they had actually survived without loss of life might have made the pain a "welcome" experience. Another masking factor might have been that the wounded, despite their gallantry and bravery, knew the pain was an automatic ticket home.

Whatever the pain-suppressing mechanisms are, they are obviously well connected to the mind and the way we view our pain.

Another interesting fact is that cultural heritage may play an important role in how we handle pain. Studies show that people of Anglo-Saxon and Northern European origin—where a stoic attitude to pain is an admired trait—actually bear pain better. In addition, research conducted at McMaster University in Hamilton, Ontario, involving 500 randomly selected households showed that women complain more than men about temporary or persistent pain.

DO WE REALLY NEED PAIN?

The honest answer is a paradox: Yes, we do, and no, we don't. You have to be able to feel pain because it is a major protective mechanism. It's your body's way of informing you that something is wrong. Without the ability to experience pain, many of us would be dead today.

Pain is still the single most common reason for seeing a physician. It's the number-one reason for taking medication. It is also the warning signal, the red flag, that says, "If you keep doing this, you're really going to hurt yourself!"

Imagine a football player who's pulled a hamstring but, since he doesn't feel any pain, continues on with his game. What's the probable end result? For one thing, he could cause irreversible damage to the hamstring; his leg will be weak and now susceptible to greater injury—a break, for example.

Okay, he doesn't feel the break when it comes, so what happens next? The fracture area will obviously be swollen, but he can't feel any pain so he goes about his everyday life for the next few days without concern. The break causes inflammation, the inflammation may become infected, and the infection could lead to gangrene. The leg, without immediate treatment, may eventually have to be amputated. In effect, without the experience of pain, this athlete could be putting his life on the line.

Obviously, not everybody is a football player. But consider the following, more down-home example that could happen if we didn't experience pain.

We all know what it feels like to attempt to drink a scalding cup of coffee; your sense of pain takes over automatically and you pull away without even thinking, because your body has been programmed to respond to pain. What would happen without that pain? You would probably continue to drink the scalding brew and severely burn your throat. This will cause inflammation and could close off your air supply. If you continued in this manner over a period of time, you'd begin to build up so much scar tissue in the throat that it would soon become impossible to breathe at all.

So you do need pain; you need pain in order to live and survive. You need pain to pull that finger away automatically when it touches a hot stove, and you even need the discomfort to tell you when you are suffering from colds and flu. It's our human version of the red stop signal.

But do you need constant pain, intractable pain, pain that nags away endlessly? Obviously not. That's why pain control, pain relief, and pain management are essential. We never want to eliminate the ability to feel pain altogether, but there is no need to endure high levels of pain continually when its presence does not serve as a danger signal. As a matter of fact, this type of pain could actually mask the protective type, so that we are unable to perceive the warning signals. That's where the Pain-Free Diet comes in.

With the correct dietary manipulation and the control of your natural pain threshold through tryptophan, you can learn to reduce pain to levels that can be lived with comfortably. What were once attacks of screamingly suicidal, head-crushing migraines can be reduced to the mere annoyance of a minor headache.

Pain is the biggest enemy of our work force, of our personal finances, and one of the largest single drains on our national economy, yet we still tend to sweep it under the carpet. Only .02 percent of the National Institutes of Health's annual budget is spent on pain research, a fact that many pain specialists find abominable.

Of course, you can continue to grin and bear your pain problems and keep on taking medications. But doesn't it make more sense to fight back with nutrition, a sensible diet, and your body's inner ability to control pain? That's what the Pain-Free Diet will teach you.

1
THE NUTRITION CONNECTION

As well as supplying energy, food plays a key role in the pain process. There are nutrients in foods from which are created the compounds that form the chain of command linking every nerve in your body with your main control center, the brain. Among these compounds are those that control how you feel, act, and perceive pain.

There are six food categories that are essential for life. In addition to water, vitamins, and minerals there are proteins, carbohydrates, and fats.

PROTEINS—THE BUILDERS

Protein is absolutely vital in your diet because it is the only source of the eight essential amino acids—the very building blocks of life. Protein is also the major source of the twelve nonessential amino acids. The term *nonessential* is very misleading because we do indeed need these amino acids. The reason we call them nonessential is that they can be synthesized within the body from the essential amino acids. In other words, if we have enough of the essential eight, we can make the other twelve.

But all proteins are not alike in their ability to provide our amino acids, and they fall into three categories: complete proteins, partially complete proteins, and incomplete proteins. It is important that we manage to achieve a good balance of all these amino acids through our protein intake.

Complete Proteins

These are protein sources that will permit growth in a child and maintain a healthy adult. If you ate only one single complete protein for the rest of your life—chicken, for example—you would still be assured of getting the essential amino acids, without any ill effects. But that would, indeed, be a very boring diet. Although we have a good variety of complete proteins, we also have other protein sources that serve not only to augment the selection of complete proteins but to provide other needed nutrient components as well.

Complete proteins include white and red meats, fish, seafood, eggs, and milk and other dairy products.

Partially Complete Proteins

These proteins include plant and vegetable forms, including beans, legumes, and nuts. They may or may not provide growth in a child, but they will maintain life in an adult when used as the sole source of protein.

These plant forms that we use as food are not as protein-rich as are animal or sea sources. It is necessary to eat much larger amounts of partially complete proteins in order to get the required amounts of the essential amino acids to synthesize the new tissue that is being formed every day.

In the adult, only maintenance amounts of essential amino acids are required because the adult needs them purely for replacement purposes. The problem with feeding a child only vegetable forms of protein is that the child literally may not be able to eat enough each day to receive the necessary amounts of essential amino acids.

It is for this reason that it is not recommended that a child of strict vegetarian parents (*vegans*) be fed exactly the same diet as the parents. A certain proportion of complete proteins should be included in the diet of the child each day—especially dairy products, not only for the protein but also for the calcium content.

Incomplete Proteins

These proteins, best examples of which are rice and corn (both lacking in essential amino acids), when used as the sole source of protein nourishment will not support life either in the growing child or the adult. In fact, ill health and eventual death will follow from malnutrition.

CARBOHYDRATES— THE MOVERS AND SHAKERS

Carbohydrates have one purpose and one purpose only: They provide glucose for energy and for the production of other important compounds made in the body. And you will see that they also play a very important role in the control of pain.

Carbohydrates include potatoes, rice, and breads—just about all of the starchy or sweet foods.

FATS—THE CATALYSTS

These are a high-density caloric source. Polyunsaturated fatty acids in fats are critical to the body for the synthesizing of other body compounds, especially hormones like prostaglandins. We tend to overeat fat in our diets. In fact, a single teaspoon of oil every day would provide all your fat needs.

A correct balance of protein, carbohydrate, and fat is crucial to the Pain-Free Diet, as you will see in the next chapter.

HOW THEY WORK

Your entire neurological system is made up of millions of nerve fibers, which run like an unimaginably complicated highway system from the tips of your fingers and toes to the control center in the brain. The main highway runs up through the spinal column in bundles of nerve fibers that come together with the brain in its stem and the thalamus. It's along these neurological highways that pain messages pass.

But also along these highways are billions of microscopic interchanges that must receive adequate amounts of the chemical substances we derive from our foods if we expect them to work efficiently. This is why specific foods are so crucial to how you feel and function. They have an indirect effect on the brain because they are needed for chemical conversions to keep the neurological freeways moving.

Among the body's most vital chemicals is a rather remarkable one as far as pain is concerned. Its name is serotonin.

THE PAIN LOCK AND ITS KEY

Serotonin is a crucial neurotransmitter in the brain, and for years scientists have been probing its importance to the whole human body. The now undeniable fact is that serotonin is the master when it comes to controlling the messages pertaining to sleep, moods, energy levels, appetite, and, yes, *pain*.

You manufacture serotonin naturally within your brain, but you need a specific nutrient from protein foods to provide the bricks and mortar to build this precious compound. This nutrient is the amino acid tryptophan.

Tryptophan is the key that turns the serotonin lock. Without adequate amounts of tryptophan in the diet, you cannot make and maintain the vital level of serotonin that is so essential to your overall good health and in controlling and regulating pain.

In addition, the entire diet is important. The proper intake of protein, carbohydrate, and fat is critical in maintaining the most beneficial level of brain tryptophan from which serotonin can then be made.

In numerous studies, scientists have identified serotonin as being the brain chemical that controls the pain threshold—the way you perceive and tolerate pain.

It is valuable here to understand exactly what the pain threshold is. The lower mark of the threshold (or recognition level) is when we first notice pain: It may be no more than a tingling sensation or minor discomfort. Certainly it is something that we can easily live with as a minor annoyance at most. The upper level of the threshold is when the pain becomes so intolerable that we must remove it immediately or continue to suffer. In the case of accident trauma, it is a violent and immediate warning that something is wrong. In the situation of chronic intractable—or long-term—pain, it is redundant, a constant reminder that we can really do without. If we can raise the high point of

the threshold, while still retaining the same lower initial
warning levels for protection purposes, we can help to eliminate much of the unnecessary chronic pain many of us
have to live with.

It is very important to recognize that pain perception and
pain tolerance are different from the pain that occurs as a
result of a definite injury or trauma (e.g., an external cut, a
broken bone, a burst appendix, stomach or intestinal ul-
ceration, etc.).

The pain process that we mostly refer to and discuss
throughout this book is the type of pain that may be "inflamed" as a result of a biochemical imbalance involving
tryptophan and serotonin.

Richard Wurtman of the Massachusetts Institute of Technology (MIT), and other researchers, showed that when animals were fed diets low in tryptophan, which brought about
resultant decreases in brain serotonin levels, the pain
threshold of these animals dropped and their sensitivity to
pain markedly increased.

Because of these studies it seemed that if we were able
to increase the amount of available serotonin in the brain,
we should be able to raise the pain threshold in patients
with chronic pain. It is just this type of biochemical imbalance that could be responsible for the extensive physical
and emotional suffering (and financial expense) that afflicts
such a great part of the American population. If we could
reduce or eliminate this type of pain, it could mean a significant leap in controlling many types of general body pain.

Our studies, initiated by Temple University's famed dental and pain researcher Dr. Samuel Seltzer, utilized carefully
controlled diets and tryptophan supplementation. They
showed that it was indeed possible to diminish appreciably,
or eliminate completely, intractable and long-lasting pain
that had been resistant to drug therapy.

Our approach, based on Wurtman's initial work, was simplicity itself—let's try to reduce pain by raising the pain
threshold!

Some of the most common sources of pain are in the

mouth and around the face and head. Because of its accessibility, the mouth is a good place to study the pain problem. Dental problems and neurological complications around the jaws and cheeks account for some of the single most savage pains known to man. It is this type of pain that can last for years.

Head, face, neck, shoulder, and even upper back pain is often caused by neurological problems among the supersensitive nerves in and around the jaw. Because of the complexity of these nerves and their closeness to our most important sense centers, it is often impossible to probe and diagnose the exact cause of these most debilitating pains.

Pain of this severity has often been described as feeling as if one's head is in a bone-crushing steel vise that clamps increasingly tighter—until you want to tear off your head to relieve the pain.

If a way of overcoming this type of pain could be found, especially one that was purely natural and didn't resort to drugs, what a breakthrough that would be!

Because it is not possible to obtain serotonin from our food (or in any supplement form), we cannot look to our diet for the direct answer. The secret of being able to boost the level of serotonin in the brain was found to be with the amino acid tryptophan, which occurs naturally in some foods. Was increasing the intake of tryptophan the key to reducing pain? It was. And in the series of studies supervised by Dr. Seltzer we were able to increase tolerance to pain significantly.

What made these studies so intriguing was that we showed that while tryptophan-boosting increased pain tolerance it did not decrease the level at which the initial perception of pain is felt. This is very important.

There are two standards of measuring pain, the first being at what level you first notice it, and the second being how much pain you can endure. One of the main concerns with raising the pain threshold was that it might also raise that all-important level where you first recognize and react to pain. This is what we call the *pain-perception threshold;*

you'll recall that pain is above all a warning, a signal that tells us something is wrong.

If we increased the threshold, people might severely damage themselves before they realize that they hurt. We had therefore utilized a natural method that allowed people to tolerate chronic pain much better, or even eliminate it altogether, without jeopardizing our early warning system.

In a real-life situation, increasing pain tolerance can mean the difference between a chronic debilitating migraine or headache and one that might just be mildly annoying or even hardly noticeable.

It's as a result of all this combined research by others and ourselves that the Pain-Free Diet, utilizing the natural powers of tryptophan, came into being as a total nutritional approach to conquer and master the problems of pain, control weight, and restore and maintain good health at the same time.

2

THE TRYPTOPHAN TIE-IN

We consider our studies on the effects of tryptophan and pain a major nutritional and therapeutic advance, and we believe millions of pain sufferers can benefit from these findings. Prior to this research, which confirmed the tryptophan-pain connection, other eminent medical and nutritional researchers had shown a variety of vital needs for tryptophan in the body.

Tryptophan is an essential amino acid. When a diet lacking in tryptophan is fed to adults, they fail to replace worn-out materials in cells, tissues, and organs. These human protein building blocks of life wear out naturally every day, so it is crucial that they are replaced. If they are not, the body begins to atrophy and waste away and the neurological systems break down.

Sufficient amounts of tryptophan are also vital during pregnancy. In laboratory experiments, when one group of pregnant rats was fed a tryptophan-deficient diet and a second pregnant group was fed a tryptophan-rich diet, the first group produced no living offspring while the tryptophan mothers gave birth to healthy litters.

Tryptophan is one of the few substances our body needs that is capable of passing through the blood-brain barrier. The blood-brain barrier is a clever system that protects the brain from absorbing chemicals that may hurt it, or that it might not need; some compounds can be absorbed through it, others cannot. It is the direct route to the brain cells themselves, and only very special selected nutrients get the golden key to enter.

It is for this very same direct-link-to-the-brain reason that tryptophan has also been found to be a critical factor in the control of mood, depression, appetite, and even some psychiatric disorders. Serotonin, as we have already discussed, is a key manipulator in brain chemistry. To have enough serotonin you need sufficient tryptophan.

Dr. O. Appenzeller of the department of neurology, University of New Mexico School of Medicine in Albuquerque, found in his research that tryptophan may play a key role in preventing migraine attacks. In some patients he found that 5-hydroxytryptophan (5-HTP), a precursor of serotonin, decreases the frequency of migraine attacks.

Dr. Richard A. Sternbach and colleagues in the Pain Unit of the Veterans Administration Hospital in San Diego, California, report that their results suggest that increased brain serotonin level causes an increase in pain tolerance. It was also noticed that tryptophan decreased depression.

Depression hits us all at one time or another, and it may well be that this is caused by an occasional lack of adequate tryptophan in the diet. Researchers in England have found that women who had become depressed during the week after giving birth had reduced levels of tryptophan in the blood, and those with the severest depression had by far the lowest levels of tryptophan.

Studies also show that premenstrual women with depression have a tryptophan metabolism disturbance. Only recently has premenstrual syndrome (PMS) been recognized as a definite biological problem for many women, not just a psychological one. These women stricken by PMS every month go through a living hell, which involves a drastic change in personality, sometimes leading to extreme outbursts of violence. PMS is now so widely recognized that it has been introduced in at least two murder trials in England as a legitimate defense for the women charged with the offenses.

It has also been discovered that postmenopausal women with depression have irregularities in their metabolism of tryptophan.

Further research indicates that tryptophan may even be superior to drugs in treating depression. In one study, two groups of depressed patients were treated, one group with tryptophan and the other with the antidepressant drug imipramine. Although both groups showed significant improvement, the tryptophan patients had little or no side effects.

Low blood levels of tryptophan have been noted in psychotics and schizophrenics. Studies at the North Nassau Mental Health Center in Manhasset, New York, revealed that sufferers of obsessive-compulsive behavior showed dramatic improvement following treatment with tryptophan.

Sleep is yet another of our most important functions in which tryptophan has now been discovered to play a major role. A study at the Maryland Psychiatric Research Center found that women who suffered from sleep onset problems were able to doze off without effort after they were given tryptophan. At the Sleep Laboratory at Boston State Hospital, insomniac patients treated with tryptophan were able to overcome their problem and sleep longer without any alteration of the all-important sleep stages.

Even the terrible tremors of Parkinson's disease have been relieved with tryptophan. In a French study, twenty sufferers of Parkinson's disease whose severe trembling could not be controlled by the traditional drug levodopa or other drugs were put on a regimen of ten grams of tryptophan daily. Eleven of the twenty found that their tremors were controlled by the tryptophan.

FEVERFEW: A STRANGE TALE FROM BRITAIN

A fascinating and slightly offbeat insight into what may turn out to be another example of the powers of natural nutritional help came from some recent research conducted in England. We think the story is worth telling because it helps to illustrate just how little we know about pain, even when an all too obvious and well-tested source of relief may have been staring us straight in the face—in this case for hundreds of years.

For centuries the folk of Britain have been taking advantage of an "old wives' tale" by chewing the leaves of a little "mum" plant for relief of migraine. Migraine and headache sufferers even put the leaves into bread and butter sandwiches and munched on them daily. The true believers vowed it was the chrysanthemum leaves that did the trick and made their migraines vanish like magic.

But not only was the little plant touted as a cure-all for headaches and migraine, it was also a panacea for sleep disorders, muscle aches, pain, and arthritic ills.

The plant, called *feverfew* by the English, has yellow and white flowers and grows wild in Europe and some parts of North America, commonly near garden walls and rivers. Its amazing properties have been highlighted in herbal textbooks going back over 400 years.

But would any serious-minded scientist get excited about a simple little plant with so-called miraculous curative powers? Well, a group of British scientists did, but it didn't come to their serious attention until an English doctor's wife gained national press publicity with her claims for it as a migraine cure. Spurred on by the demand to know more about feverfew, scientists at King's College in London began studies involving its users, while researchers at Chelsea College began to look into its pharmacological secrets.

Dr. E. Stewart Johnson of King's College, who is also

honorary research director of the City of London Migraine Clinic, conducted a study of 300 feverfew users. The scientist was astonished to discover that seven out of ten subjects using feverfew reported that their migraine attacks were less frequent, were less painful, or had disappeared altogether. All of these migraine sufferers had tried and failed to find relief from over-the-counter medications and prescription drugs. Another surprise was the incidence of pleasant side effects, such as less pain from their arthritis, or symptoms of a tranquilizing nature, less muscular tension, and more restful sleep. "We have to consider this remarkably high success rate as a breakthrough in the treatment of migraine," Dr. Johnson admitted later.

Meanwhile, biochemists at the University of London made an astounding discovery when they analyzed the chemical composition of feverfew. They discovered chemicals never before seen in plants. But because of patent possibilities the researchers are keeping their findings a closely guarded secret. However, in reviewing some of the researchers' published documentation we found a clue to what one of those mysterious chemicals might be.

The researchers reported that among the plant's fascinating chemicals were ones that were found to either enhance or suppress known substances in the human body, including histamine, prostaglandins, and 5-hydroxytryptamine. What's 5-hydroxytryptamine? Yes, you might have guessed it . . . serotonin! Could one of those mystery chemicals be tryptophan? At the moment that is strictly a hypothesis; only time will tell.

A NATURAL WONDER DRUG?

Well, is tryptophan the newly discovered natural wonder drug of our age? All the data on tryptophan is not yet in, and probably won't be for some years. But we feel it's useful to know what other pioneering work is going on with this wondrous amino acid, and we'll discuss this in more detail in Chapter 14.

Our primary concern with tryptophan is its unique function in the control of pain. But as you can see from the previous examples of other research in the field, the Pain-Free Diet may have some remarkable additional health benefits for people suffering from other problems as well as pain.

THE CARBOHYDRATE CONNECTION

Let's get right down to the action of tryptophan and explain how it works, and why your diet is critical to its utilization.

In pioneering studies at MIT, Dr. Richard Wurtman and his wife, Dr. Judith Wurtman, made a dramatic discovery by showing that carbohydrate is a key factor in the production of serotonin because of its action in helping to get tryptophan to the brain. And it is here that we find another major dietary key to tryptophan and pain.

Carbohydrates are starchy and sweet foods. When they are eaten they release insulin into the bloodstream, and insulin is an aid to tryptophan's journey to the brain. This is why the Pain-Free Diet is higher in carbohydrates, lower in fat, and balanced in protein compared to the normally high-protein, high-fat, traditional American diet.

But isn't there a contradiction here? Why reduce protein when we know the only source of tryptophan is from protein? As the Wurtmans showed, eating larger amounts of protein actually lowers brain tryptophan levels as more of the competing amino acids are present to occupy space that could belong to tryptophan.

In order for the tryptophan to get into the brain it must first cross the blood-brain barrier. To do this it is not a matter of simply passing through tiny holes, like sand through a sieve. There is an actual transport mechanism to which the tryptophan becomes attached, and in this fashion it is ferried through from the outside of the barrier to the inside, where it is free to mingle with the blood that circulates throughout the brain. The carrier is a complicated chemical system with which we needn't concern ourselves.

Tryptophan, however, has to compete with five other amino acids for space on this transport system. The competing amino acids are phenylalanine, tyrosine, valine, leucine, and isoleucine (these are called large neutral amino acids, or LNAA). Under the best of circumstances tryptophan would have a one-in-six chance of getting onto the transport system and gaining entrance to the brain.

The problem is compounded by the fact that the level of tryptophan in foods is much lower than that of LNAAs, and therefore, it has a still harder time competing with the larger numbers of LNAAs for the limited space available.

Contributing to this entire process is insulin. When you eat carbohydrate of any kind, insulin is secreted into the bloodstream in order to control the levels of glucose in the blood and ensure that too much of it doesn't get into the brain. Insulin is the body's glucose "minder." This is all happening at the same time that tryptophan and the other competing amino acids are being loaded into the bloodstream as the protein content of your meal is being digested.

In addition to helping the body control the level of sugar (glucose) in the blood, insulin also has another job that makes it a friendly ally of tryptophan. It actually acts something like the bloodstream's traffic cop and distributes the LNAAs by channeling the amino acids into tissue cells— thus reducing the number of them heading for the brain and, therefore, decreasing the competition that tryptophan will encounter when it gets to the blood-brain barrier. But why doesn't tryptophan get swept along with the LNAAs?

Tryptophan has a special "pass." The LNAAs travel in the blood as free amino acids; they are not bound or bonded to any other substance, but tryptophan is. It is bound to albumin in the bloodstream. If we use the analogy of insulin as the traffic cop, we see that he directs most of the LNAAs into the tissue cells but when he spots the tryptophan with the albumin he recognizes it as having a special pass and waves it onto the direct route which will take it to the blood-brain barrier.

Eating more tryptophan-rich foods doesn't ensure that more tryptophan reaches the brain, because of the fierce competition from the other amino acids at the blood-brain barrier.

What's the solution? As well as having balanced protein in our diet, we can also increase carbohydrate intake, which ensures that more insulin is present. Dr. Richard Wurtman made these significant discoveries in his research involving tryptophan and serotonin and their unique relationships to the food chain.

He explains the tryptophan connection and its anomalies this way: "When we eat protein-rich foods, we consume relatively small amounts of tryptophan (usually less than 1 percent by weight) but much larger amounts of the other neutral amino acids. Hence, the greater the amount of protein in the diet, the more difficult it is for tryptophan to enter the brain.

"Paradoxically, the single meal that most effectively elevates brain tryptophan (and serotonin) is the one that completely lacks protein." A candy bar might therefore elevate brain tryptophan better than a glass of milk.

Dr. Wurtman adds, "Of course, chronic consumption of a tryptophan-poor diet will reduce the amount of the amino acid present in the whole body, including the brain."

And what follows in a tryptophan-deficient diet is that no matter how satisfactory you make the surroundings for ideal tryptophan transportation, the initial lack of it in the blood system is not going to boost serotonin production.

The last major nutrient group that can hinder the successful transportation of tryptophan to the blood-brain barrier is fat. When digested, fat yields compounds called fatty acids. These fatty acids do not travel as free chemicals in the bloodstream—they too bond together with albumin and have the pass that gives them free travel past the insulin traffic cop.

Fatty acids are so unruly that if they do travel free, they can cause serious damage. The body has a natural setup to protect itself against this, but it can work against tryptophan. Because of the danger of freewheeling fatty acids running around the bloodstream, the body gives preference to dealing with them by ensuring that they attach to albumin first, before tryptophan does. In fact, if tryptophan has already bonded with albumin and a free fatty acid comes along, the tryptophan will be bounced from the albumin, which then bonds with the fat. Tryptophan is left without a vehicle home.

So, you can see now why it is so important not to have too much fat in the diet, and it is therefore essential that it be carefully controlled.

To sum up, by following the Pain-Free Diet, with its balanced protein, increased carbohydrate, and lowered fat content, you are creating a superhighway to the brain for tryptophan. You are going to be getting the maximum potential of tryptophan in optimum amounts, especially with the addition of tryptophan supplements to the diet. It's probably easier to see now how you can get a natural handle on your pain problems.

"But aren't carbohydrates one of the most fattening foods? After all, I'm trying to lose weight as well as pain!" you might exclaim. That's a question we are always asked. The breakthrough research providing the explanation was conducted by Dr. Judith Wurtman at MIT.

Dr. Wurtman found that many of us have a craving for carbohydrates, and this is quite natural. We have what she calls a carbohydrate hunger. And she discovered that the only way to turn off the carbohydrate hunger is by feeding it with carbohydrates. That's logical. But aren't we in danger

of eating more and more carbohydrate to satisfy that craving, and getting even fatter?

The truth is actually the opposite! Dr. Wurtman's experiments, which she describes in detail in her book *The Carbohydrate Craver's Diet*, showed her that only a small
amount of carbohydrate is often all that's needed to quell
carbohydrate hunger. The key here is that serotonin throws
the switch which turns off carbohydrate hunger. It's the
perfect combination. With the right balance of carbohydrate
and protein, tryptophan heads for the brain and increases
the serotonin level. When this level is sufficient, serotonin
initiates the message saying "enough carbohydrate."

Now you can see that when you eat carbohydrates together with a balanced amount of protein you have the
essential ingredients together not only to relieve pain but
to turn off carbohydrate hunger as well.

CLINICAL TESTS OF TRYPTOPHAN

Clinical studies carried out at Temple University School of
Dentistry showed that by creating the most beneficial dietary conditions for serotonin production (*i.e.*, a properly
adjusted protein, carbohydrate, and fat diet) and adding supplements of tryptophan to the diet to boost its potential,
pain levels were significantly reduced.

An initial study was performed by Dr. Seltzer, chairman
of the department of endodontics, on a group of selected
volunteers who were free from pain. The object of this study
was to determine whether the pain-tolerance level could be
increased.

The subjects were tested for both their sensitivity and
tolerance to pain. To do this, a novel method was introduced
by Dr. Seltzer: a tooth pulp stimulator. This small battery-
operated device is essentially a probe that transmits a small
electric current from its tip. By means of a control knob,

the current can be varied, producing a range of response from a tingling sensation to actual pain.

The probe was placed against a tooth, and by slowly increasing the current flow the individual being tested would indicate two points: when the current was first felt (the pain-perception threshold, normally a tingling sensation) and when he or she could no longer tolerate the level of induced pain (the pain-tolerance level).

All the test subjects (thirty in all, twenty-six males and four females) were rated for both their perception threshold, and for their pain-tolerance level. These values were noted for all thirty, and then the subjects were divided into two groups, fifteen subjects in each.

In a double-blind procedure, fifteen of the subjects received tryptophan while those in the second group were given identical-looking cellulose placebo capsules (an inert substitute that looked like the tryptophan capsules). Each tryptophan capsule contained 250 milligrams of the amino acid, and the volunteers were instructed to take two capsules six times a day: at breakfast, midmorning, lunchtime, midafternoon, and a double dose before retiring. Each of the subjects either received 3 grams of tryptophan or the placebo each day for seven days.

Vitally important to this research was ensuring that the tryptophan was given the optimum conditions to do its job. Each subject was put on the tryptophan-boosting high-carbohydrate, low-fat, balanced protein diet, identical to the expanded version of the diet you'll find in this book.

On the eighth day of the study the subjects were retested with the pulp stimulator and their scores recorded. In the tryptophan group there was a significant increase in pain tolerance, some even doubling their ability to endure pain. Also extremely important was that they showed no change in their pain-perception threshold. The subjects were able to first perceive the transmitted current at the same levels they did originally, before the introduction of tryptophan supplements.

In the fifteen subjects who did not take tryptophan there

was a slight improvement in their ability to tolerate pain, but it was statistically insignificant. This could possibly be attributed to the beneficial conditions created for the natural food-supplied tryptophan action through their improved diet. Their pain-perception thresholds also remained the same as their previous readings.

The subjects were also asked to report on any side effects they felt. Amazingly, the tryptophan group reported not only feeling more rested and relaxed but in much better spirits. Mood elevation was reported by ten of the tryptophan subjects. This was very exciting because it helped confirm previous clinical research by others where mood elevation was reported in the treatment with tryptophan of patients suffering from depression. The fact that some subjects also felt more rested after having received the tryptophan echoes previous reports that tryptophan can induce better-quality sleep and also produce a sedative effect.

Since then, exciting results with tryptophan-boosting have been observed in hundreds of pain patients. It was felt that these important human observations could mean relief for millions who have to suffer continual or recurring pain each day of their lives.

This new knowledge, regarding the optimum utilization of tryptophan, is the very essence of the Pain-Free Diet. Is there really any reason for anybody to continue suffering when you have the ability right at your fingertips to conquer pain?

3
FOODS THAT EAT YOU

There are certain foods that can cause havoc with your daily diet. They can not only produce severe bouts of pain, but they can also upset the natural nutritional pain balance, and may even have been responsible for throwing you off previous weight-loss plans.

No, these are not poisons or toxins; they are ordinary foods that you encounter every day and may be one of the causes of your persistent pain problem. That's why we need to look at these offenders and consider eliminating them first before starting the Pain-Free Diet.

You'll even find these foods listed in the menus of some of the best-selling so-called diet books. If you've ever tried a diet program that caused you discomfort, pain, and possibly nausea, and gave you a general feeling of malaise, it could very well be that these offending foods were the cause.

These nutritional pitfalls are one of the least recognized causes of pain by most people outside scientific and medical circles. We've termed them *the foods that eat us;* they fight back all the way through the digestive process, not all of them using the same method of attack. The discomfort and pain they produce can range from severe migraines and headaches to upset stomachs and muscle aches. Some severe reactions to these edibles include serious breathing distress and dermatological eruptions of the skin.

The biggest problem with this class of foods is they don't react uniformly from one person to another, and that makes them very difficult to identify as pain culprits. We know what they are: foods like cheeses and chocolate, flavorings like licorice, and drinks that range from coffee to champagne. Even some vitamin supplements can cause problems.

For example, two people may be enjoying clam chowder together in a restaurant. Later in the evening one of the diners complains of having a headache and feeling slightly nauseous, while the other feels perfectly okay. They put it down to the meal, rationalizing that the sick one must have hit on a bad clam. In fact, the stricken diner may have an allergic reaction to clams, or may have recently developed one. That's another problem with these offending foods; their ill effects are often transient.

Another major problem is that it may not be the food itself, but a flavoring or coloring that has been added, in either its production or its cooking. A common example is the popular addition of monosodium glutamate (MSG) as a flavor enhancer in Chinese cooking.

At Temple University we see a good many people who suffer from head and neck pain and other body aches and pains. In two years of studying the food-pain link, Temple researchers are now able to predict that at least 5 percent of head- and neck-pain sufferers will have their problems traced directly back to substances in their diets. Many of the subjects who took part in these studies were able to obtain relief by simply eliminating the particular foods that were "eating" them. We must stress, however, that not all these foods affect all people the same way.

So far we have managed to identify twenty-five separate pain syndromes that are caused directly by substances we eat or drink. Some of these act as vasoconstrictors, which means they narrow the blood vessels. And when this happens in the head and neck, the buildup of pressure inevitably leads to migraines, headaches, neck pain, and aches that can go right into the shoulders and upper back.

Others act as vasodilators. What happens here is that the blood vessels swell, and this also leads to pain, especially when it involves the blood vessels in the brain.

We have seen chronic-pain patients at their wits' end come to us for help. They've suffered repeated bouts of agony, many have been to countless physicians with their problems, and yet they still cannot find any relief. With a bit of detective work we can often trace the cause directly back to specific foods they eat.

The significance of being able to recognize these offending dietary substances is that the treatment is often as easy as just omitting them from their daily diets. In the case of vasoconstrictors and vasodilators, the symptoms show up quickly after the ingestion of the substance, sometimes as soon as twenty or thirty minutes later.

Because of this short time span it makes it an ideal problem for you to analyze yourself. It's easy for anyone to pinpoint a possible culprit in their diet if shortly after a meal they come down with the gremlins. By removing the suspect foods on a selective basis, it's possible to isolate the offender and remove it from your diet completely.

Here's an example: If you have just had a sandwich, a cup of coffee, and a bar of chocolate and you come down with a headache shortly after, it's a good guess that one or more of them could be the problem. Next time you try the same combination, eliminate the chocolate. If you still get the follow-up headache, it's pretty certain chocolate is not your problem. Next time, keep the chocolate and omit the coffee. If that doesn't work, it's most likely to be something in the sandwich. You simply keep eliminating and substituting until the malefactor is discovered.

If you utilize this technique, you can get off to a flying start with the Pain-Free Diet because you've already isolated the most likely violators. Here are some of the more common offenders.

monosodium glutamate (MSG)
licorice
smoked fish
bologna
salami
pepperoni
bacon
frankfurters
corned beef
canned ham
cheeses (especially aged cheddars)
canned figs
pickled herring
chopped liver
yeast
pods or broad beans
Marmite (trade name)
chocolate
coffee (not decaffeinated)
tea
champagne
red wine (especially Chianti)
herbal teas
alcohol
beer
nutmeg
seafoods (certain ones)
over-the-counter medications (certain ones)
vitamins (certain excesses)

With this handy reference table it's easy to spot the substances you might commonly eat or drink. Now we'll take them individually and explain why they might have an adverse effect on your particular body makeup.

CHEESES, FIGS, PICKLED HERRING, LIVER, CHAMPAGNE, YEAST, BROAD BEANS, COFFEE, CHIANTI, MARMITE, BEER: These all contain a substance called *tyramine*. Tyramine activates the noradrenaline system and causes vasoconstriction to occur.

Natural and aged cheeses, particularly the cheddars, are very high in tyramine content. Amphetamines combined with cheeses and alcohol can cause highly elevated blood pressure resulting in immediate headaches. Tyramine is also a suspect in triggering migraine attacks.

SMOKED FISH, BOLOGNA, SALAMI, PEPPERONI, BACON, FRANK-FURTERS, CORNED BEEF, CANNED HAM: These all contain nitrate and nitrite compounds. These chemicals are used in the curing process to preserve the foods and prevent botulism. They are also used to impart a pinkish color and give a cured flavor to meats. But unfortunately for some, nitrates and nitrites act as vasodilators and cause migrainelike headaches and jaw and neck pain. It's commonly known as the *hotdog headache*. As little as five milligrams of sodium nitrite can produce a headache in susceptible individuals.

MONOSODIUM GLUTAMATE: Monosodium glutamate can be put in a category all by itself because it can appear in a wide variety of foods, too many in fact to mention.

Its most common use is in Oriental cooking as a flavor enhancer, and this has led to the term *Chinese Restaurant Syndrome*. It's an uncomfortable attack that can result in nausea, headache, undue sweating, and palpitations.

A special word of warning here for people who take diuretics. You should be especially cautious of MSG because it can produce a condition known as transient hypernatraemia (excessive sodium in the blood).

The symptoms are:

- a sudden tightening of the muscles of the face and throat, numbness;
- constriction of the muscles of the back and neck;
- a feeling of pins and needles in the mouth;
- a feeling of nausea, dizziness, and even giddiness;
- sweating and flushing of the face;
- severe pain in the jaws, neck, and shoulders;
- a tight bandlike headache;
- palpitations and weakness.

Although these symptoms can cause severe distress, recovery usually occurs within thirty minutes of the onset of an attack.

MSG can be found commonly in canned soups, potato chip products, gourmet seasonings, some dry-roasted nuts, certain processed meats, instant gravies, and TV dinners.

LICORICE EXTRACT: Fortunately, this is not a common problem in the United States because most licorice used in candies and drinks is artificial.

But for some, genuine licorice can cause hypertension, facial edema, and severe muscle weakness, pain, and tenderness.

Licorice extract is eaten as a confection and is used as an expectorant, as a treatment for ulcers, and as a flavoring additive to some drugs and alcoholic drinks.

CHOCOLATE: Chocolate has been described as one of the most common dietary triggers of migraine headaches. Although it does not contain tyramine, it has a similar effect and causes the release of vasoconstricting noradrenaline from the heart and blood vessels. Recent research also indicates that chocolate can increase the risk of migraine attacks for someone already susceptible to them.

COFFEE AND TEA: Caffeine acts as a vasoconstrictor. People who drink five or six cups of coffee a day are ingesting some 1,000 milligrams of caffeine.

Caffeine decreases the flow of blood to the brain by constricting the cerebral blood vessels—but, conversely, this effect may cause striking relief for sufferers of headaches associated with hypertension, and certain types of migraine.

But when caffeine consumption is stopped, a throbbing headache appears in one quarter of high-caffeine consumers within eighteen to twenty-four hours. This effect can also be seen in the "weekend headache syndrome," when people who are used to regular coffee breaks during their workweek begin to suffer caffeine withdrawal symptoms.

Caffeine also has other side effects. Sleep disturbances are common, including delayed onset of sleep and an increase of night awakenings. Mood swings are also associated with heavy caffeine intake.

It is very important to know that the drinking of coffee, tea, or soft drinks containing caffeine causes a significant and long-lasting increase in the amount of fatty acids released into the blood from our fat stores. These fatty acids, of course, bring about a decrease in the amount of tryptophan that can arrive at and penetrate the blood-brain barrier. Try to eliminate, or reduce to a minimum, your caffeine intake.

So, how much caffeine is considered heavy? A dose of 250 milligrams is considerable, yet 20 percent to 30 percent of Americans consume more than 500 to 600 milligrams per day, and 10 percent sip over 1,000 milligrams per day. To estimate your own consumption check the following list. Remember, some soft drinks and colas contain caffeine.

1 cup brewed coffee	75–155 mg
1 cup instant coffee	86–99 mg
1 cup tea	60–75 mg
1 cup decaffeinated coffee	2–4 mg
1 bottle cola drink (12 oz)	30–65 mg
1 cup of cocoa	2–40 mg

HERBAL TEAS: Not too much is known about herbal teas, but their popularity is growing as they are sold over the counter not only as drinks but as psychoactive drugs, cathartics, and diuretics.

The effects of herbal teas are varied, and because there are so many different varieties it's difficult to predict them all. But they can range from nausea and headache to severe dryness of the mouth and throat. One herbal tea made from burdock plants is reported to cause blurred vision, dry mouth, inability to void, as well as bizarre behavior and speech.

A number of herbs are used in, or as, teas, including juniper, catnip, jimsonweed, wormwood, hydrangea, and lobelia.

NUTMEG: As well as being an additive to foods and desserts, nutmeg is also used for the relief of stomach upset and flatulent colic. But nutmeg also has some bizarre side effects, including euphoria and hallucinations. It's believed that these effects from the dried kernels of the seeds of the nutmeg tree may be linked to the chemical they contain called myristicin—a compound remarkably similar to the hallucinogenic mescaline.

Nutmeg can cause headaches and liver damage. Even small amounts (*i.e.*, two ground nutmegs in a glass of water or soda) can cause headaches, cramps, and vomiting.

SEAFOOD: The problem with seafoods, particularly mussels, clams, oysters, and scallops, is that they can contain a potent neurotoxin called saxitoxin. Some people are particularly sensitive to saxitoxin—even to the point of death.

Regular seafood eaters who constantly complain of headaches and muscle cramps should look at their seafood platters as a potential cause of their difficulty.

Saxitoxin blocks neurological signals to the muscles and can cause temporary paralysis. Because saxitoxin can be not only agonizing but fatal, the following symptoms are listed. Medical attention may be an immediate necessity.

- burning and tingling of the face, tongue, gums, and lips
- spreading of numbness to the arms and legs and especially the fingertips
- progressive paralysis. This can result in increased difficulty in breathing and even complete respiratory failure.

OVER-THE-COUNTER MEDICATIONS: Many cold preparations, painkillers, and even curatives like Bromoseltzer contain caffeine. Even some prescription drugs do. When you start to total your daily intake of caffeine, don't overlook these otc medications that may be having an adverse effect on you.

Here's a list of the caffeine content of some common preparations:

```
otc stimulants ................................. 100 mg
otc cold preparations ........................ 30  mg
Bromoseltzer, Anacin, aspirin compound..... 32  mg
Empirin Comp, Midol, Cope, Easy-Mens..... 32  mg
```

Vanquish .... 60 mg
Excedrin .... 66 mg
Pre-Mens .... 30 mg

If you are at all unsure about the caffeine content of any otc medications, check the containers for listings or ask your pharmacist.

VITAMINS: Because of the boom in the sale of vitamin supplements there has also come the problem of regularly overdosing on them. It happens easily, especially now with the availability of so many multivitamin pills, boosters, and the so-called megavitamins. Beware! Abuse of vitamins can also cause you painful problems.

Vitamin D. Excessive ingestion of vitamin D supplements can cause nausea, anorexia, weakness, severe headaches, and gastrointestinal disorders.

The recommended daily dietary allowance (RDA) for vitamin D is 400 international units (IU).

Vitamin A. While any excess of vitamin A can cause problems, the introduction of high-potency vitamin pills and capsules makes it even easier to take too much. The RDA for vitamin A is 4,000 IUs for women and 5,000 IUs for men. For children from six months to ten years old the suggested ration is between 2,000 and 3,000 IUs per day.

The toxic dose for vitamin A is regarded as some 50,000 IUs a day over a period of at least a year. This may sound like an awful lot, but people actually do take these amounts.

Constant excesses of vitamin A can cause headaches, thickening and yellowing of the skin, and increased susceptibility to disease.

Niacin. This is a vasodilator. The usual RDA for niacin is about twenty milligrams a day. For some people niacin, even in small doses, can cause face flushing and burning, and tingling around the face, neck, and hands. This is a normal effect and shouldn't be a matter of concern. But constant overdosing of niacin will definitely cause these uncomfortable effects and may include headaches.

ALCOHOL: Alcohol is a vasodilator, and it can also depress and alter central vasomotor centers. This can produce headaches and cluster headaches in susceptible individuals.

Remember that as well as the usual alcoholic beverages we are used to drinking, alcohol appears in significant quantities in cough medications, some nonprescription expectorants, elixirs, tonics, liquid vitamins, and even your regular mouthwash.

The best way not to let certain foods "eat" you is to recognize which they are, consider how often you eat them, and try to remember any times when you may have been able to connect a particular incidence of pain to the eating of one of these substances. Then start the process of elimination.

The cause of your pain may very well be your own favorite foods. But take heart, you may be able to return to them later after you've eliminated them from your diet and "detoxified" their effects. New research shows evidence that once the offending foods have been eliminated and their painful symptoms have disappeared, it may be safe to return to eating them in small doses spaced widely apart (a week or more) without any of the previous effects. This is a matter about which you will have to make your own personal decision.

LACTOSE INTOLERANCE—A VERY SPECIAL MESSAGE ABOUT MILK

Just about everybody drinks milk, but for some of us it can have unwanted side effects. This problem occurs mainly as we grow older and may even start in the twenties. As we age, our bodies begin to tolerate milk less than they used to. This condition is called lactose intolerance (the inability to tolerate this sugar in our body) or lactase insufficiency (a shortage of the enzyme lactase, which is responsible for digesting the milk sugar, lactose).

As babies, we manufacture the enzyme lactase in the intestinal tract. This enzyme is responsible for digesting (splitting) the disaccharide sugar, lactose, into the constituent monosaccharide sugars that make up lactose—glucose and galactose.

Lactose is only found in milk and milk by-products, and in no other food source. Although both of its constituent sugars are used for energy, galactose is especially important to the baby because it is used in the formation of nerve tissue. We do make galactose in our body, but the lactose in the milk (whether in human breast milk or other animal milks) helps to augment the amount made by the baby at this particular time of major growth of every component in the body.

As we grow older the lactase enzyme begins to disappear. Humans are, in fact, the only mammals that continue to drink milk after weaning—no other animal does this as a natural function of its eating habits. Because of this evolutionary reason for not requiring the enzyme, the body simply begins to phase out its production. The body naturally assumes that we are not going to be drinking any more milk once we pass the stage of needing it and therefore won't be needing the lactase to digest the lactose sugars.

But milk and dairy products are still important to us as the most concentrated source of food calcium. The decline in lactase production as we age doesn't occur suddenly and may never decline in many individuals. The tendency is there for this enzyme to gradually diminish, so we must accept that we are all subject to this process. The problem is that the diminution of lactase production in our bodies may be so gradual that we don't realize it. If you are a milk drinker, you may never recognize the connection between the symptoms that result and their cause.

What are the symptoms? Over a period of time, even many years, we can experience gurglings and rumblings in the gastrointestinal tract, increasing flatulence, and diarrhea. As these effects become more severe and troublesome, we seek advice and help. But even physicians may not be aware of the true cause.

What's actually happening is that when the lactose is not digested in the small intestine by the action of lactase, the sugar cannot be absorbed. The now undigested sugar continues on its trip and into the large intestine. It's here where the troubles begin. The resident bacteria in the bowel are able to digest the lactose—and they start to have a ball on this welcome new source of food. As a result, the metabolic by-products of the gastronomic overactivity cause all of the symptoms that we now recognize as *milk distress syndrome*.

There is, however, a solution. Milks that are free from lactose—or have the lactose predigested—are now available at most dairy counters. If you cannot immediately spot them, ask a sales assistant for help in finding them.

Moreover, yogurt and buttermilk will not affect the lactase-deficient individual because the bacteria used in the culturing process have already digested the lactose.

Lactase, both in tablet form and liquid, can be purchased from pharmacies and health food stores for adding to your own milk supplies. A few drops of the liquid lactase added to a carton or glass of milk are enough to do the trick. The tablets can be carried with a person and swallowed prior to eating a meal that may contain milk, for example, in a restaurant. Both methods are extremely effective.

A tip to recognize milk that has had its lactose removed is that it tastes slightly sweeter than untreated milk.

4

A NUTRITION OVERVIEW

Built into the survival blueprint for all life is the innate recognition that food is essential; it is necessary to get it in sufficient quantity in order to live. It is only in the past century or so that we have come to recognize that the quality as well as the quantity of food is important.

Diseases like scurvy and beriberi were conquered only when it was finally realized that these fatal conditions were not caused by something alien in our bodies, something that had to be gotten rid of (like curses, or, later on, infectious bacteria), but that there was actually something missing that needed putting into our bodies. It was from the research into these pathological conditions that the dawn of realization occurred. And from that came our knowledge today for the needs of such substances as ascorbic acid (vitamin C) and thiamine (vitamin B_1).

Maybe you like to eat Italian food, or possibly French, Oriental, or Mexican. What all these foods have in common is their chemical constituents: what they are composed of.

In all the foods that exist in the world (it's worth remem-

47

bering that all foods have previously been other forms of life) there are, at present, approximately fifty-one individual chemicals absolutely essential for our survival. Because not many people like to think of ingesting chemicals, we refer to these instead as nutrients.

Properly selected foods provide the majority of nutrients we need: We are actually capable of making one fifth of those nutrients—provided we have the required starting material, or ingredients, in the diet. More about this later on.

The fifty-one nutrients are divided into six categories. These we have already mentioned in Chapter 1, but now we will go into more detail.

The essential six are proteins, fats, carbohydrates, vitamins, minerals, and water. And the water is not just to slosh the other five around so they can be dissolved (we have some amazing gastrointestinal acids to do that). Water is an actual chemical compound that is just as essential to life as the other nutrients are. As a matter of fact, in order of priority, water comes in second only to oxygen for life support.

We can remain alive without breathing for only minutes; without water life is measured in days, with air and water but without food possibly weeks, depending on the stores of nutrients that are already available within the body. But it is only a matter of time before the effects of nutrient deficiency become apparent.

From the nutrients in foods are created the compounds that form the chain of command which links every nerve in your body with your pain-control center, the brain. Among these compounds are those that control how you feel, act, and perceive pain.

PROTEINS

Protein is absolutely vital in our diet because it is in protein that we find amino acids. There are twenty different kinds of amino acids. These amino acids are divided into two groups: essential and nonessential amino acids. Essential amino acids—all eight of them—cannot be manufactured in our bodies and we *must* obtain them from the foods we eat.

But all proteins are not alike in their ability to provide the twenty amino acids. Proteins, then, are identified as to their ability to do the job that they are meant to do, which is, after all, the important task of keeping us alive.

So, proteins fall into the three categories we outlined in Chapter 1: complete, partially complete, and incomplete.

Complete proteins contain all of the essential and non-essential amino acids. Partially complete proteins may not contain all of the essential amino acids, or they may be deficient in the amounts of one or more of the essential amino acids. Incomplete proteins lack essential amino acids.

Do we know how much amino acids or how much protein we need to consume each day? The answer is yes. Extensive nutritional studies have shown that the amount of amino acids required for all of our biochemical functions in the body is contained in about .5 gram (one fifty-sixth of an ounce) of protein per pound of body weight. In the RDA table (which you will find later in this chapter) you will see that the recommended protein intake for an average-size adult woman is 44 grams (or 1.6 ounces per day), while for an adult man the amount goes up to only 56 grams (2 ounces) of protein per day. This does not mean that two ounces of meat are all the adult male requires (meat contains fat and water in addition to protein). What it does mean is that the total amount of protein contained in two 3-ounce meat patties (at 7 grams of protein per 1 ounce of meat: $7 \times 6 = 42$ grams protein) constitutes just about the entire day's allowance for a woman. Three of the same type of meat patty will do it for a man.

The amount of protein being recommended amounts to from 10 to 15 percent of the total daily caloric intake. The average American consumes at least twice this amount, if not more. This is an important fact, and we'll discuss it in more detail later.

CARBOHYDRATES

The major form of carbohydrates that we use for food—the starches—is made up of only one chemical compound, glucose. Carbohydrates have one major purpose: They provide glucose for energy and for the manufacture of other important compounds made in the body. As we have already pointed out, carbohydrates play a very important part in the control of pain. Carbohydrates include just about all of the starchy or naturally sweet foods, including potatoes, rice, and grains.

Two other souces of carbohydrate in our diet are sucrose (table sugar) and lactose (milk sugar), which is only found in breast milks. Both sucrose and lactose contain sugars other than glucose, but in the body even these sugars are changed into glucose.

How much carbohydrate should we include in our diet? There hasn't been any specific amount determined by scientific nutritional studies. But we can calculate it, and this method works out quite well in providing the body with the correct amount sufficient to take care of the energy needs and the other specific purposes to which the body puts glucose to use.

Since we've already stated that protein should constitute from 10 to 15 percent (fat you will later find to be 30 percent of the total daily caloric intake), carbohydrate should amount to from 55 to 60 percent. Now, this doesn't mean candy and cake. What we are referring to are complex carbohydrates: These are starches composed of hundreds of thousands of glucose units in straight and branched chains linked together. When these glucose units (molecules) are grouped in these large numbers, the starches made up of such big chains don't even taste sweet.

We usually wouldn't describe raw potatoes as sweet, but when we cook these starchy foods some of the glucose can hydrolyze (break free) from the rest of the chain—and this glucose can taste sweet. This is exactly what happens, for example, when carrots are cooked.

FATS

We don't need the fat we get from our foods at all! To be more precise, we do not require the fat content of food. We can make as much fat as we need—and even more than we need, as many overweight people know. But what we do need from fats and oils are the compounds called polyunsaturated fatty acids, which we cannot make in our bodies. Just as with the amino acids, we must get them from our dietary sources. Although meat contains polyunsaturated fatty acids, they do not originate with animals; what the animals have of them comes from certain plant foods they eat. So, we get the fatty acids we need either from the plant foods directly or from the animals that eat the plants.

The problem with eating animal meats, like beef, is that in addition to getting the fatty acids we require we also get much, much more of other kinds of fatty acids that are made by the animal's own body—the saturated fatty acids. These we definitely do not need! Usually we have far too much of that kind of fat, and not only do we take in what is contained in the meats but we also make our own as well. Our personal production generally comes from the excess carbohydrate we take in, in addition to the fat we eat.

The type of fatty acids that we do need—the polyunsaturated fatty acids—come from oils in such plants as corn, peanuts, safflower, and soya, and in cold-water fish.

Unfortunately, we tend to overeat fat in our diets. As we have noted, the amount of essential polyunsaturated fatty acids needed to provide for all our daily needs could be contained in just one teaspoonful of safflower oil. It's worth knowing that all the proteins contained in the complete protein category (meats, poultry, seafood, dairy products, and eggs) contain fats. It's therefore impractical even to try to plan a fat-free diet. What we can do, however, is cut down on those foods rich in saturated fats.

Do we know how much fat we should eat daily? Not as accurately as we do protein. But all the studies so far indicate that the fat we take in each day should not exceed 30 percent of our total caloric intake.

The fat intake of the average American has been calculated at 45 percent or more. The American Heart Association has attributed the high level of cardiovascular heart diseases, and the resultant mortality from them, to the high intake of fat. Death from heart disease is today the nation's number-one killer. Second is death due to cancer. And the American Cancer Society has declared that a high proportion of breast cancer and cancer of the bowel is due to the excess intake of fat in the American diet.

VITAMINS

Vitamins are what the body uses to process the amino acids, the fatty acids, and the glucose. They are absolutely necessary to life. We can take the essential amino acids apart like tinker toys and use the parts to make the nonessential amino acids. But it is rare we can do the same with any of our other food substances to make the necessary vitamins. Again, our primary source of vitamins should be the foods we eat.

Vitamins are needed only in very tiny amounts, and our requirements are measured in quantities ranging from milligrams (one twenty-eight thousandth of an ounce) down to micrograms (one twenty-eight millionth of an ounce). But these amounts, tiny as they are, are absolutely necessary to make up the enzyme systems that are the very basis of life.

The last vitamin to be discovered was vitamin B_{12} in 1949. Since that time no other compound has been isolated that meets the condition of being absolutely essential to life— regardless of the number of substances being sold today that have the letter B as part of the label.

Vitamins fall into two categories, fat-soluble and water-soluble. Whereas we can build up stores of fat-soluble vitamins within our tissues, water-soluble vitamins have to be replaced on a daily basis because they are depleted through fluid loss by the body.

Nutrition studies have given us a good idea as to the amounts of these substances that we need each day. The recommended dietary allowances (RDAs) for all vitamins are:

vitamin A	5,000 IU
vitamin E	30 IU
vitamin D	400 IU
vitamin K	70–140 mcg
vitamin C	60 mg
folic acid	0.4 mg
thiamine	1.5 mg
riboflavin	1.7 mg
niacin	20 mg
vitamin B_6	2 mg
vitamin B_{12}	6 mcg
pantothenic acid	10 mg
biotin	100–200 mcg

FAT-SOLUBLE VITAMINS

Vitamin A

Source: eggs, milk, butter, green and yellow vegetables, carrots, liver

Function: maintaining skin and mucous membranes, production of visual pigment

Deficiency result: poor tooth and bone development, night blindness, mucous membrane and skin disruptions

Benefit: protection against skin diseases, bolstering of the immune system, possible anticancer activity

Toxicity: greater than 50,000 IU a day over extended periods of time. Symptoms are muscle and joint pain, fatigue, weakness, headache.

Alternative: beta-carotene (pro-vitamin A). We can safely build up stores of beta-carotene in the body, which will then convert to the more potent vitamin A when needed.

Vitamin D

Source: butter, fish oils, egg yolk, liver; also synthesized in the skin from the action of sunlight

Function: normal bone formation and maintenance; calcium metabolism

Deficiency result: poor bone formation, deformities and degeneration, rickets

Benefit: treatment of osteoporosis (weakening of the bone structures with the result of increased risk of fractures) and rickets

Toxicity: 4,000 or more IU per day

Vitamin E

Source: green and leafy vegetables, grains, seed oils, butter, liver

Function: healthy cell-membrane construction, antioxidant, prevents cell-membrane damage

Deficiency result: not clear at the present time

Benefit: treatment of vascular disease (especially concerning the brain), stress, some skin disorders, and possibly in aging and cancer

Toxicity: none reported

Vitamin K

Source: green leafy vegetables

Function: normal blood clotting

Deficiency result: disruption of blood-clotting factors. Also antibiotics can kill bacteria in the intestine that are responsible for producing vitamin K.

Benefit: maintains the fine balance between the anticoagulant and clotting powers of the blood

Toxicity: none reported

WATER-SOLUBLE VITAMINS

Vitamin C

Source: fruits and vegetables

Function: necessary for synthesis of hormones, collagen synthesis (the glue that holds body cells together), wound healing, resistance to infections, use of iron

Deficiency result: scurvy, many problems with the skin and inability to heal, gum inflammation, anemia, general lethargy and weakness

Benefit: treatment of immunological deficiencies, allergies, inflammation

Toxicity: Excessive doses can be detrimental in an unusual way. The body will create appropriate enzyme levels necessary to maintain proper levels of vitamin C. When excess quantities are ingested (for some people this could be amounts over 1,000 mg a day) and the person suddenly stops taking C cold turkey (*i.e.*, ran out of it on a Thursday and intends to buy more on the weekend), the enzyme work force that has been built up to cope with excess amounts of C doesn't know to stop and continues to rid the body of all the C it finds. The result: what is called *rebound scurvy*, which can occur within a day or two with all the symptoms of initiating scurvy—bleeding gums, bruise marks, etc. Can also result in intestinal discomfort.

Vitamin B₁ (thiamine)

Source: yeast, wheat germ, grains, legumes, pork, liver

Function: carbohydrate metabolism

Deficiency result: anorexia, weakness, inability to coordinate muscular movements, abnormal nervous sensitivity, wasting away of tissues, mental confusion, pain

Benefit: promotes normal function of the nervous system

Toxicity: none reported

Vitamin B₂ (riboflavin)

Source: grains, eggs, vegetables, dairy products, yeast, liver

Function: fat and carbohydrate metabolism, energy production

Deficiency result: skin inflammation (cracked lips, inflamed tongue)

Benefit: treatment of skin and inflammatory diseases, promotes good vision and healthy skin

Toxicity: none reported

Niacin

Source: meat, fish, poultry, dairy products, yeast, peanut butter

Function: carbohydrate and fat metabolism, energy production, tissue respiration

Deficiency result: weakness, irritability, anorexia, skin and gastrointestinal lesions

Benefit: proper utilization of carbohydrate for energy; promotes healthy skin, nerves, and digestive tract; aids digestion and normal appetite

Toxicity: can produce harmless flushing, headaches, and nausea

Vitamin B$_6$ (pyridoxine)

Source: meat, fish, liver, vegetables, grains, legumes

Function: essential in protein metabolism, fatty acid metabolism, conversion of tryptophan, red blood formation

Deficiency result: anemia, skin disorders, irritability, muscle twitching, kidney stones, nervous dysfunction

Benefit: treatment of anemia

Toxicity: some reports of nerve damage following long-term high levels of intake

Vitamin B_{12}

Source: milk and milk products, eggs, cheese, meat, poultry, seafood

Function: normal development of red blood cells, maintenance of nerve tissue

Deficiency result: anemia, neurological problems, dementia

Benefit: treatment of pernicious anemia and neurological disorders

Toxicity: none reported

Folic Acid

Source: legumes, green leafy vegetables, liver

Function: amino acid metabolism

Deficiency result: anemia, weakness, red tongue, diarrhea

Benefit: treatment of anemia, metabolism of food proteins

Toxicity: none reported

Pantothenic Acid

Source: meats, milk, egg yolks, whole grains, liver, legumes

Function: energy metabolism

Deficiency result: fatigue, weakness, depression, sleep disturbances

Benefit: proper energy metabolism

Toxicity: none reported

Biotin

Source: yeast, egg yolks, liver, vegetables, kidney, milk

Function: synthesis of fats, amino acid metabolism, glucose storage as glycogen in the liver and muscle cells

Deficiency result: dermatitis, fatigue, depression, muscular pains

Benefit: all of the above

Toxicity: none reported

MINERALS

Most people are aware of the effects of lost salt, and it's the first mineral we commonly replace. But there are other important ones, too.

We have known for at least one hundred years that there are mineral substances in the body which are necessary for life. Because of the large amounts of calcium in the bones we knew this element was necessary for structural purposes and was thus part of the skeleton and other protective formations of the body—like the skull, which protects the brain.

We learned that iron was an important part of the red blood cell, the function of which is to carry oxygen to each and every cell in our body.

Iodine was discovered to be part of an important hormone, thyroxine, which is made in the thyroid gland. If we don't get our required amount of iodine, the thyroid glands (located on both sides of the trachea) strive to grow larger in the mistaken notion that if they do increase in size they will be able to make the required thyroid hormone.

This is what gave rise to the condition known as *goiter*, which afflicted so many Americans in the "Goiter Belt"— the midwestern part of the United States that is equidistant from the Atlantic and Pacific oceans. Since seafood constitutes the best source of iodine and early food transportation systems made it impossible to store and ship such perishable commodities, those parts of the country that were denied fresh seafood suffered from a lack of iodine. It was for this reason that iodized salt came into being; adding iodine to such a commonly used food item ensured the intake of this needed element.

Today we hear of the importance of such minerals as copper and zinc and chromium. We are familiar with copper in electrical wires, and chromium is for car bumpers. What do these minerals have to do with our health?

Since all life arose from what was once a primordial soup containing all the elements dissolved from the earth's crust, it's not too surprising that after billions of years the chemical reactions that were successful in bringing about the life process would still be part of living systems today. And it is these biochemical reactions that use the calcium, iron, zinc, copper, and chromium that are still retained and are part of mammalian biochemical systems—which include our own.

The essential minerals are generally divided into two categories: first, the minerals that are required in amounts more than ten milligrams per day, and second, the trace elements that are required in smaller amounts.

The recommended daily dietary allowances for adults are:

```
potassium .........  1.9–5.6 grams (1,900–5,600 mg)
sodium.............  1.1–3.3 grams (1,100–3,300 mg)
chloride ...........  1.7–5.5 grams (1,700–5,500 mg)
calcium ............   .8–1.0 grams   (800–1,000 mg)
phosphorus........   .8–1.0 grams   (800–1,000 mg)
magnesium.............................  300–350 mg
iron (men) ......  10 mg....... (women).......  18 mg
zinc .................................................  15 mg
```

manganese................................ 2.5–5.0 mg
copper .... 2.0–3.0 mg
fluoride.................................... 1.5–4.0 mg
molybdenum............... .15–.2 mg (150–200 mcg)
chromium................... .05–.2 mg (50–200 mcg)
selenium.................... .05–.2 mg (50–200 mcg)
iodine .... 150 mcg

5
WHAT'S WRONG WITH THE AMERICAN DIET?

Americans may be the best-fed people in the world, but we're paying a high price for our faulty food habits. In a national study conducted by the Department of Agriculture, only half of the 7,500 families surveyed met the recommended dietary allowance for protein, calories, and other essential vitamins and nutrients. The rest failed to meet the RDA standard for one or more of these categories.

At the same time, chronic diseases have been on the increase, with millions of people suffering from migraines, backaches, and arthritic problems, just to name a few.

The Pain-Free Diet offers a lifetime eating plan that will change not only your attitudes and your health but the quality of your life as well.

And whether you want to stay healthy, lose weight, or simply eliminate pain problems, just about everyone can benefit by including the Pain-Free Diet in their lives.

There is a growing national recognition that one special type of balanced diet is far more beneficial than any of the others—a balanced protein, increased-carbohydrate, low-fat

TABLE I

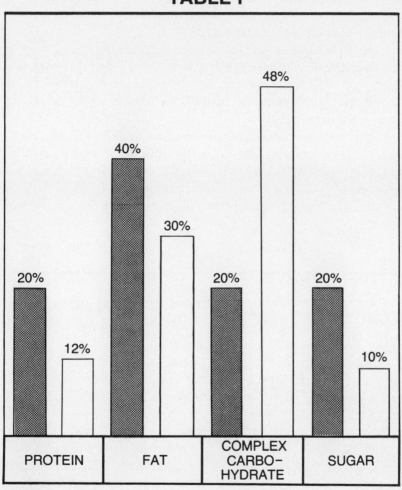

diet. Ask the American Heart Association, the American Cancer Society, the National Institutes of Health which type of diet they recommend!

To help begin to focus in on your present dietary strengths and weaknesses, please study the table (Table I) on page 63. In it, you will see how a basic American diet compares to the dietary goals recommended by the federal government and health agencies.

Later in this chapter and the next we will be showing you exactly how to calculate your own personal dietary needs, whether you intend to lose weight, maintain it, or gain a few pounds—and all on a diet that provides the optimum conditions for the wonderful pain-free aspects of tryptophan.

WHY IS PROTEIN NECESSARY? THE BALANCE THAT PAYS DIVIDENDS

You already know quite a bit about the chemical composition of protein from previous chapters. Now let's look more closely at some of the body functions for which it is necessary.

Protein is essential for the formation of all body tissues, including bones, nails, and hair. It also constitutes the makeup of blood, enzymes, and hormones, and builds the antibodies that protect us from diseases. In order for your body to operate at its peak efficiency level, it's necessary to take in a daily supply of top-quality protein.

But as current studies of dietary habits show, most of us take in too much protein. And too much of a good thing can be just as harmful as not enough.

We've already shown that unless the protein intake is controlled, the tryptophan will not work properly. Once the balance gets out of kilter, a high-protein diet will simply make us feel worse instead of better.

How Much Protein Is Too Much?

Let us examine how the body handles the nutrients that we take in—not just protein, but carbohydrate, fat, vitamins, and minerals.

All of these nutrients are subject to the actions of the liver, which can be thought of as a factory. An easy way to understand what's happening is to visualize a conveyer belt. You are standing at this conveyer ready to start working. Also alongside you, and across from you, are other people who are also ready to begin working at their assigned tasks. At one end of the conveyer belt are parts that have to be assembled by the workers so that at the other end of the belt a finished product emerges. Rather than toasters or vacuum cleaners, however, products coming from the liver's assembly line can range from protein prothrombin (necessary for blood coagulation) to more than 80 percent of the globulins that assist us in combating infection and disease.

Just as in any conveyer belt system, the ability of the workers to put parts together and work well in harmony depends on how fast the conveyer belt is moving. If the parts aren't put onto the conveyer belt fast enough, the workers stand idle and the finished products are delayed or simply not produced.

In a company that must produce a certain output each day in order to stay in business, such inefficiency might well cause the firm to fail. It's the same in our human factory. In the body all of the compounds that are produced are absolutely essential in order to maintain an optimum health status. If these compounds aren't made at a specific rate—the prothrombin for the blood-clotting mechanism, the enzyme that is essential for a specific function, the insulin necessary for proper carbohydrate metabolism, or a chemical unit that must be produced as a part for another product on a different assembly system in the body—then we are in big trouble.

If these products (compounds) are not made at the proper

rate, then other manufacturing plants within the body that perhaps depend on these units begin to suffer—and our over-all health starts to deteriorate.

Just as the assembly line fails if the parts aren't coming fast enough, too rapid a supply will also cause the workers problems. Remember, once you have swallowed your dinner and it has all been digested, there is no way to control what happens to this material. If there is too much of any par-ticular commodity—protein or fat, for example—the body must now contend with it, whether it needs it or not. All this must be accomplished in the cellular factory regardless of whether it can afford to take the time and effort away from other important duties in maintaining the human machine.

Our systems were designed to handle all the nutrients that we digest at a certain optimum rate. If we abuse this year after year, the factory loses its ability to maintain homeostasis (the state of keeping everything in the proper balance throughout the entire body's mechanisms). When this begins to happen, the disorders that result are reflected in a departure from general good health, and there is really no telling finally how many aspects of health will suffer!

The one particular condition that we are addressing is the imbalance (disorder) that brings about pain: chronic, in-tractable, around-the-clock pain that no drug can correct. This biochemical imbalance in the body's mechanism can be corrected only by carefully adjusting the flow and content of the biochemicals (nutrients) involved in this particular system.

We know we need these nutrients, we know in what ratio they should be to each other, but do we really know *how much* of all these nutrients we need?

With protein we have a fairly accurate answer provided by nutritional research. Presently, the amount that will pro-vide for just the right amount of protein to yield the desired amounts of amino acids to be loaded onto our human con-veyer belt is about .5 gram of complete protein per pound of desirable existing body weight. This is equivalent to between 10 and 15 percent of the total daily caloric intake.

Here's how to calculate the approximate amount: Assume a caloric intake of approximately 2,000 calories per day. That's about the national average. Let's use the lower protein figure of 10 percent since the calculations will be easier. 10 percent of 2,000 calories is 200 calories' worth of protein.

Since protein will yield 4 calories per gram (one twenty-eighth of an ounce), divide the 200 calories by 4 to give the value of 50 grams of protein. This means that 50 grams of protein is the allowance for the entire day.

To give you some idea of how 50 grams of protein translates into food, we'll again take the typical 3-ounce beef patty. The 3-ounce patty contains 20 to 25 grams of protein. Two of these beefburgers, then, contain all of your protein allowance for the entire day!

But don't panic. You won't have to split two meat patties into little pieces to spread among breakfast, lunch, and dinner—we'll explain later how you are to handle your protein intake. You'll also find the same for carbohydrates and fats.

Protein Calories Do Count

Foods high in protein can actually add up to a lot of calories, even when compared to carbohydrate-rich foods such as pasta, rice, and potatoes. Take, for example, a three-ounce steak compared to a cup of spaghetti with tomato sauce. Would you guess that the steak has less calories? That both would be about equal? Or that the spaghetti contains more calories? If you figured the steak has more calories than the spaghetti, you are already becoming a smart eater. The steak actually contains about 500 calories, compared to the cup of spaghetti with tomato sauce at a mere 200 calories.

And while protein has long been considered the dieter's

friend, burning up faster than either fats or carbohydrates, recent research now shows this may not be so.

In an exacting study done at the University of California at Berkeley, the caloric benefit of a high-protein diet was compared with one that was more balanced. The results showed no significant difference. On a similar theme, scientists at the University of Virginia compared laboratory rats on a high-protein diet with rats given the same number of calories but less protein. The weight gain in the first group of animals was higher than that of the controls who were fed much less protein and more carbohydrates.

Your Optimum Protein Allowance

According to carefully explored studies by the National Research Council (NRC), it has been possible to compute a daily protein allowance that the body needs to maintain optimum physical health.

In the following table (Table II), based on a person's weight,

TABLE II

Recommended Daily Dietary Allowance for Protein*
(assuming average height)
These are average figures and may not reflect exactly your own personal computations

	Age	Weight (lbs)	Protein (gm)	Protein (oz)
MALE	11–14	99	45	1.58
	15–18	145	56	2
	19–22	154	56	2
	23–50	154	56	2
	51 +	154	56	2

	Age	Weight (lbs)	Protein (gm)	Protein (oz)
FEMALE	11–14	101	46	1.6
	15–18	120	46	1.6
	19–22	120	44	1.55
	23–50	120	44	1.55
	51 +	120	44	1.55

Information supplied by the Food and Nutrition Board, National Academy of Sciences–Nutritional Research Council, Washington, D.C.

you can get an idea of the RDA for protein as recommended by the NRC.

If you do not find your weight listed in the table, refer to the formula in Table III to find your optimum protein level. If you are planning to lose weight, simply substitute your ideal weight for the current weight, as indicated in the chart.

Once you've found your recommended protein allowance, record the number here _____ for a handy reference marker (you're going to refer back to it later).

TABLE III

Computing Your Daily Protein Allowance

Your current weight × .5* = Total grams of protein per day

For example:

130 lbs × .5 = 65 grams

.5 refers to grams of protein per pound of ideal weight.

CARBOHYDRATES CAN HELP YOU LOSE WEIGHT: TURNING ON YOUR BODY'S TURNOFF SIGNAL

Carbohydrates are not only the key for shedding aches and pains—they can also be the magic ingredient for losing pounds as well. Sounds strange? Well, remember back to the section on carbohydrate hunger and being able to turn it off! Carbohydrates, found in sweet and starchy foods, are converted by the liver into glucose, which, you'll recall, is the main energy source for the body.

At the same time this is happening, the body produces the hormone insulin to keep the sugar in the blood at a normal level. By eating carbohydrates together with the right amounts of protein, the insulin that has been released into the bloodstream then paves the way for the blood to carry the tryptophan into the brain and boost the amounts of available serotonin.

Once the serotonin levels are sufficient, there's an automatic turnoff of the body's carbohydrate craving. And the brain sends the signal back to the body saying, "Enough! I'm full!"

Instead of falling victim to hunger pangs—the greatest downfall of many dieters—you'll find you are no longer hungry, and you'll be able to go happily until the next meal without the least bit of discomfort.

Fast Foods—An Uneasy Solution

As the Pain-Free Diet recommends a high carbohydrate intake, and most fast foods are high in carbohydrate, does this mean those quickie, calorie-laden meals can stay on the menu?

Unfortunately, eating fast foods can be a bad dietary practice. Fast foods are not only fast to produce but even quicker to consume. Most require little chewing before swallowing.

Eating too rapidly defeats a natural mechanism that all of us are blessed with to help us control the amount of food we take in.

This natural diet control depends on chewing food thoroughly and swallowing at a much slower pace than we do with fast foods, and even most snacks. When the food arrives more slowly, our body has a chance to judge just how much is entering and permit our appetite control mechanism to work—to let us know when we are getting to that point when we really do not need any more food. It won't tell us whether the food was the right or the wrong kind—just how much of it went down.

The function of the appetite control is compromised, however, by swallowing the food so rapidly that it doesn't register properly. It's usually only when we actually feel stuffed that we say we've had enough. At this stage, unfortunately, we are well beyond the "enough" peak: We've reached the engorgement level. Can you just imagine what these amounts of nutrients are doing to the body's conveyer belt system?

The tendency to gulp food results in continually getting down more food before the body has the opportunity to realize it has overeaten. Or, to be more truthful, it has been made to overeat by what we have done to override the very control our body depends on to adjust the amount of each meal.

In short, fast foods are not to be recommended as a nutritional lifestyle!

Consummate Carbohydrates

When we refer to the beneficial effects of carbohydrates in the Pain-Free Diet, we are talking about the natural complex carbohydrates, starches and sweets found in fruits, vegetables, and cereal grains. These are higher in fiber and more filling than refined sugars.

These foods provide a distinct advantage to the dieter in

that they are bulky and take longer to chew, thus filling the stomach and small intestine without the dieter having to consume too many calories.

FRIENDLY FATS

Fats are friends of sensible nutrition, but they also should not be abused. As you have already learned, a little fat goes a long way in providing the essential processes for life.

Fats also serve other functions; they help insulate us from heat, cold, and trauma, and they store the fat-soluble vitamins A, D, E, and K.

Additionally, fats and oils accentuate most of the flavors in foods. And invisible fats can be found in practically all processed food products. Most fats supply our need for the essential fatty acids (linoleic, linolenic, and arachidonic), which are not produced naturally in the body and must be supplied by an outside source. Because we need only the essential fatty acids, anything else just piles on pounds. For example, do you really want to inherit from the cattle all the excess pounds of fat they had to put on to produce the tasty beef we consume? No, because we humans don't need it—but that's what can happen when we consume too much fat contained in our meat products.

Because fats are digested more slowly than carbohydrates, they promote a longer-lasting sense of fullness. However, as the name implies, fats are the most fattening of the three nutrient groups—weighing in at nine calories per gram, more than an equal part of either protein or carbohydrate.

The American Heart Association has now warned that a high-fat, high-cholesterol diet is a key link to heart disease. The American Cancer Society also reports an undeniable connection between this type of diet and breast cancer and cancer of the colon.

Another thing is for sure—a diet high in fat will most certainly pack on the pounds.

6

LEARNING TO EAT SMART

In order to experience a pain-free lifestyle, regulate your weight, and create optimum health, you first have to be a smart eater. This chapter will show you how.

Many people start diets with lots of good intentions. But the minute they reach their weight goal their motivation wanes, and the pounds simply roll right back into place.

With the Pain-Free Diet, you won't need willpower, the adhesive that helps us stick to most traditional diets. But you must be willing to make a permanent commitment, because the changes we are going to show you should best be followed for your lifetime.

Although this may sound impossible at first, *you can do it!* And you'll want to do it all the more once you realize how wonderful it can make you look and feel.

You've already found out what's wrong with what you have been eating; now you're ready to discover what's right for the proper dietary maintenance of your health and weight.

To get started on the Pain-Free Diet immediately, you'll be given fourteen days' worth of meal suggestions at four different calorie levels. Simply choose the level that suits your dietary needs (this you'll find explained later in the chapter). In the meantime, you can get busy designing your own personalized diet plan.

At the beginning, your new eating habits may take some getting used to. But before you know it, you'll get to be such an expert on the foods and their nutritional values that the whole process will become second nature.

As many participants in the Pain-Free Diet have already learned, eating right can be its own reward. Once you have successfully incorporated your new eating habits into your lifestyle, you'll also be able to make adjustments for that every-once-in-a-while urge to cheat.

Best of all, you'll not only have a whole world of food to choose from, you'll also feel marvelous—maybe for the first time in your life. You'll find that you will never want to return to your old eating habits again.

HOW MANY CALORIES A DAY DO I NEED?

To Maintain Your Present Weight

All you need to do is multiply your present, or desired, weight by your activity level.

Your activity level is determined by the number of calories it takes to maintain a pound a day. If your lifestyle is fairly sedentary, stick to 12 calories; use 14 if you are moderately active; and 16 if you are very active.

Translated into numbers (for a person weighing 130 pounds) it would look like this:

$$
\begin{array}{ll}
130 & \text{(present or desired weight)} \\
\underline{\times\ \ 12} & \text{(activity level)} \\
1{,}560 & \text{(total daily calorie intake)}
\end{array}
$$

If your goal is to maintain weight, record your total daily calorie level here: _____.

To Lose Weight

One pound of fat is equivalent to 3,500 calories. To lose one pound per week, you will need to eat 3,500 less calories per week—or 500 calories less each day.

To lose two pounds a week, you would need to decrease your daily calorie intake by 1,000. (*Note:* There are no short-cuts to slimness. And a weekly weight loss of more than two pounds is not recommended in the interests of good health.)

You've seen (in our example) that it takes approximately 1,560 calories a day to maintain a weight of 130 pounds. In order to lose ten pounds and reach a goal of 120, you need to reduce your daily caloric intake by 500 (1,560 calories minus 500 calories) to a level of 1,060 calories for the next ten weeks.

If you are planning to lose weight, write your estimated daily dietary intake here: _____.

Finding Your Ideal Weight

Now for the good news! You may think you are overweight, but the chances are that you are not!

Many of us have a distorted picture of our own bodies, the one we see every day in the mirror. It's similar to the phenomenon known by every person who's ever appeared in front of a television camera, but this time your own mind is the camera. Any television director, cameraman, actor, or actress will tell you that your image on television or film will look a good eight to twelve pounds heavier than you really are. There's no magic to this; it's just a trick of optics. If you ever meet a well-known television or film celebrity, who you've always considered had the perfect body, you'll suddenly be surprised to see how much thinner he looks in person.

It's also known among nutritionists that most people who believe they are "unreasonably" overweight are actually not. You might well benefit by losing a couple of pounds or so, but any more may even be unhealthy for you as an individual, and may cause more stress than it's worth.

The enlightening news today is that being a little overweight is healthier than being underweight. In studies at Johns Hopkins University, Dr. Maria Simonson, director of the famed Health, Weight, and Stress Program in Baltimore, Maryland, has come to the conclusion that we worry too much about excess weight: "The simple truth in this country is that concern about weight reduction has been carried too far. We have become slaves to a 'desirable weight' set of tables devised by the life insurance companies. These tables were formed to simply predict mortality rates, not health.

"What the statistics do is make most of us feel inadequate, unattractive, and unacceptable if we exceed their limits. For years we have struggled, starved, and slimmed to conform to them."

Because of the pressure from Dr. Simonson and other health professionals the Society of Actuaries and the Life Insurance Medical Directors of America have revised their tables in a welcome upward direction.

The National Heart, Lung, and Blood Institute reports that standard weight tables produce more stress for Americans who consider themselves overweight than inflation. And the National Institutes of Health report that thin people have a higher mortality rate than persons of average weight.

In Massachusetts a long-term epidemiological study of women age 40 to 69 years old discovered that the highest death rate was among the thinnest and the most obese women, while the lowest was among the broad range of women in the intermediate weight ranges.

A recent industrial study of men in their fifties who were 25 to 32 percent above the "desirable" weight ranges showed they lived longer than either their thinner or fatter counterparts.

It is now generally agreed in the nutrition field that the old guidelines for "normal weight" should be increased by about ten pounds on average for women and some fifteen to twenty pounds for men.

You can find your most beneficial weight by checking the weight charts we have included, which take into account our new understandings of health and ideal weight.

HOW THE DIET WORKS

The diet is based on an exchange system that will allow you great flexibility in putting together your own interesting, easy-to-live-with meals. In it you'll be able to mix and match foods from the basic food groups, as well as a number of tasty snacks. What you choose is really up to you as long as you stay within the required allowances necessary to maintain your daily protein, carbohydrate, and fat levels.

You already know:

- your recommended protein allowance,
- your daily calorie intake,
- the Pain-Free Diet guidelines for healthy eating (*i.e.*, 12 percent protein, 58 percent carbohydrate, and 30 percent fat).

Now you are all ready to put it together. So, let's get out paper and pencil and begin.

CHART I

Your Ideal Weight Chart[†]

MALES

height**	small	medium	large
		frame size*	
		pounds	
5'	101–122	103–129	109–134
5'1"	104–129	109–134	113–140
5'2"	110–135	114–141	119–146
5'3"	114–141	119–146	123–152
5'4"	120–147	124–153	129–158
5'5"	122–153	129–158	133–164
5'6"	126–159	134–165	139–170
5'7"	130–165	139–170	143–176
5'8"	134–171	144–177	149–182
5'9"	138–177	148–182	153–188
5'10"	142–184	152–189	158–195
5'11"	146–189	156–195	163–200
6'	151–196	160–201	167–207
6'1"	161–201	166–207	171–212
6'2"	169–208	174–213	178–219
6'3"	174–213	178–219	183–224
6'4"	179–220	184–225	188–231
6'5"	184–225	188–231	193–236

*Finding your frame size: Measure the circumference of the wrist on the hand that you write with.

MEN: Small—under 6 inches; medium—6–7 inches; large—over 7 inches.

**Measure height in stocking feet.

†Source for chart: Dr. Maria Simonson, Director of the Health, Weight, and Stress Program, Johns Hopkins Medical Institutions, Baltimore, Maryland.

CHART I

Your Ideal Weight Chart†

FEMALES

height**	frame size*		
	small	medium	large
		pounds	
4'8"	86–96	93–103	98–118
4'9"	88–99	95–106	100–121
4'10"	90–102	97–109	102–124
4'11"	92–105	99–112	105–127
5'	93–111	100–117	106–128
5'1"	95–117	101–122	107–130
5'2"	100–122	104–128	109–133
5'3"	104–128	109–133	113–139
5'4"	109–133	113–139	118–144
5'5"	113–139	118–144	122–150
5'6"	118–144	122–150	127–155
5'7"	122–150	127–155	131–161
5'8"	127–155	131–161	136–166
5'9"	131–161	136–166	140–172
5'10"	136–166	140–172	145–177
5'11"	140–172	145–177	149–183
6'	145–177	149–183	154–188
6'1"	150–182	154–187	159–194
6'2"	155–186	159–193	164–200

*Finding your frame size: Measure the circumference of the wrist on the hand that you write with.

WOMEN: Small—less than 6 inches; medium—6–6.5 inches; large—over 6.5 inches.

**Measure height in stocking feet.

†Source for chart: Dr. Maria Simonson, Director of the Health, Weight, and Stress Program, Johns Hopkins Medical Institutions, Baltimore, Maryland.

EIGHT EASY-TO-FOLLOW STEPS TO DESIGNING YOUR OWN DIET

1. Write down your daily caloric intake here: _____ .

2. Write down your recommended protein allowance here: _____ .

3. Next, to find out how many grams of fat you should be eating, follow this simple two-step formula:

a) multiply your daily caloric intake by 30 percent.
For example: 1,560   (total calories)
                   × 30%   (daily fat RDA)
                   468   (total calories)

b) convert this figure to grams:
divide 468 calories by 9 (there are 9 calories in every gram), which equals 52 grams.

Record your daily allowed fat intake here: _____ .

4. To compute your carbohydrate allowance, use the same procedure with the following numbers:

a) multiply your daily caloric intake by 58 percent.
For example: 1,560   (total calories)
                   × 58%   (daily carbohydrate RDA)
                   905   (total calories)

b) to convert your calculation to grams:
divide 905 calories by 4 (there are 4 calories in every gram of carbohydrate), which equals 226 grams.

Record your daily allowed carbohydrate intake here:
_____ .

5. Now take a sheet of paper and set up a chart similar to the one illustrated in Table IV.

TABLE IV

A	Prot	Fat	Carb	Cals
	--------------------*grams*--------------------			

BREAKFAST

1. _____ ____ ____ ____ ____
2. _____ ____ ____ ____ ____
3. _____ ____ ____ ____ ____
4. _____ ____ ____ ____ ____
5. _____ ____ ____ ____ ____
6. _____ ____ ____ ____ ____

MIDMORNING SNACK

1. _____ ____ ____ ____ ____
2. _____ ____ ____ ____ ____
3. _____ ____ ____ ____ ____

LUNCH

1. _____ ____ ____ ____ ____
2. _____ ____ ____ ____ ____
3. _____ ____ ____ ____ ____
4. _____ ____ ____ ____ ____
5. _____ ____ ____ ____ ____
6. _____ ____ ____ ____ ____

MIDAFTERNOON SNACK

1. _____ ____ ____ ____ ____
2. _____ ____ ____ ____ ____
3. _____ ____ ____ ____ ____

DINNER

1. _____ ____ ____ ____ ____
2. _____ ____ ____ ____ ____
3. _____ ____ ____ ____ ____
4. _____ ____ ____ ____ ____
5. _____ ____ ____ ____ ____

| (continued)   **TABLE IV** |

A	B			
	Prot	Fat	Carb	Cals
	----------------------*grams*----------------------			
6. _____	____	____	____	____
7. _____	____	____	____	____
8. _____	____	____	____	____
LATE-NIGHT SNACK				
1. _____	____	____	____	____
2. _____	____	____	____	____
3. _____	____	____	____	____
	____	____	____	____
		TOTAL		

Beginning with Part A, write down a sample break-fast that you would normally eat during the week (just pick one day from the week to get an idea of your eating pattern). Do the same for lunch and dinner. And don't forget to include the snacks.

6. Once you've recorded your meals in Part A, you're ready to calculate Part B. Turn to the exchange lists in the following chapter and fill in the food equivalents that are listed.

For example, you will see that one slice of bread is equivalent to 13 grams of carbohydrates, 2 grams of protein, and 70 calories. Write these values on your sheet, and do the same for every food item. Once you complete the list, add up your totals.

Most likely, you'll find that your present eating habits are way off base compared with the daily allowances you've just computed for the Pain-Free Diet. To meet these new requirements, you're going to have to redesign your meals and portions to get your diet back in line.

7. This is where you can start getting creative. Begin with your fats first. Try to trim off some of the excess you've been eating. For example, instead of heaping a pat of butter on your morning toast, cut the portion in half. If you are used to using a lot of butter in your food preparation, see where you can decrease the amount or switch to nonfat items. Then do the same for your carbohydrates, and finally the protein.

   Keep working back and forth, trading food choices until you're able to establish a reasonable balance in all the categories and they match up as closely as possible with your ideal dietary requirements.

8. If you find that your calorie totals are on the low side and you need to add some foods, try to make up the difference first with carbohydrates.

   Remember, whether you are planning to lose weight, maintain it, or even gain a few pounds, the foods you eat are the key to achieving your goal. Nature has given us a wide variety of delicious choices to pick from that are not only nutritious but also low in calories and good for our health. The trick, which the Pain-Free Diet teaches, is how to put this all together for a lifetime of optimum physical health.

Note: You can also use the menus—see Chapter 9—as a guide, or you can use them directly for fourteen days, and combinations of them for future daily and weekly meal plans. *The choice is yours:* Calculate your own or utilize the preprepared menus. Remember, the value of calculating your own meals is that you have at your fingertips the power to create any meal for any occasion, and it will always be in perfect nutritional balance.

7

THE PAIN-FREE DIET EXCHANGE LIST

Here are the exchange lists of foods that make the Pain-Free Diet the most interesting, nutritious, tasty, zesty, and easy-to-assemble diet you've ever experienced.

Thousands of wonderful dishes can be prepared from the following food listings, and the numerous combinations literally make your menus limitless. They can range from simple on-the-run snacks to four-course gourmet dinners. Just let your imagination run away with all the mouth-watering possibilities.

All you have to do is follow the guidelines, and then start mixing and matching the foods for your own customized diet. We suggest that you keep paper and pencil handy to make notes of your favorite food combinations for future reference.

In Chapter 9 you will find sample menus for fourteen days at four different calorie levels: 1,000, 1,500, 2,000, and 3,000 calories a day. You can either utilize these menus for the first two weeks on the diet or treat them as a handy guide for developing your own.

Remember, unlike other diet plans there is no barrier to limit the inventiveness of your Pain-Free Diet plan.

GENERAL GUIDELINES

1. The basic food groups are divided into six sections. Any food may be exchanged for any other food on the same list if the appropriate amounts are used. There is also a seventh list that includes some additional foods, beverages, and sweets that you may also wish to incorporate into your dietary regimen.

2. Be sure to use the amount specified for each serving. The measurements are expressed in terms of the eight-ounce measuring cup, the standard teaspoon or tablespoon, or in terms of common food portions.

The abbreviations used in the tables are as follows:

sm	small
med	medium
lge	large
sl	slice
oz	ounce
lb	pound
tbsp	tablespoon
tsp	teaspoon

The serving sizes are based on the following standard measurements:

1 cup	8 fluid ounces or 16 tablespoons
2 tablespoons	1 fluid ounce
1 tablespoon	3 teaspoons
1 pound	16 ounces or 453.6 grams
3.5 ounces	100 grams

3. Use your own judgment to determine what is small, medium, or large. If anything is unclear, call it large. In the long run it's better to overestimate.

   Similarly, estimating the size of a 4-oz piece of meat can be done by weighing it or making a sight judgment of the portion based on the package content. (For example, if the package says 4 ounces, you know that ¼ of the amount present equals an ounce.)

4. To calculate the number of calories in a specially made-up recipe that's not on the list, such as meat loaf or a homemade soup or stew, look up each ingredient used in the final product, total the amount, and divide by the number of servings for a portion count.

5. Become a label reader. Be aware of all the ingredients you're eating, especially when it comes to dietetic foods.

6. When a particular food is not listed, select the closest equivalent food; the selection will be close enough to provide an approximate content of the three nutritional categories and their total caloric value.

1: MEAT EXCHANGE LIST

One exchange of lean meat contains approximately 7 grams of protein, 2 grams of fat, no carbohydrate, 55 calories.

BEEF: baby beef (very lean), chipped beef, chuck, flank steak, tenderloin, sirloin, plate ribs, plate skirt steak, round (bottom, top), all cuts rump, spareribs, tripe, ground beef (low fat content)............................ 1 oz
LAMB: leg, rib, loin (roast and chops), shank, and shoulder .... 1 oz

PORK: (whole rump), center shank, shoulder............ 1 oz
HAM: smoked (use only center of slices), boiled .... 1 oz
VEAL: leg, loin, rib, shank, shoulder, cutlets............ 1 oz
LIVER: beef, fried.. 1 oz
POULTRY: meat of chicken (without skin), turkey,
    Cornish hen, guinea hen, pheasant .... 1 oz
FISH: any fresh or frozen.................................... 1 oz
    canned salmon, tuna, mackerel, crab, lobster .... ¼ cup
    clams, oysters, scallops, shrimp .... 5 indiv. or 2 oz
    fish sticks................................... 1½ (plus ½ bread)
    sardines, drained .... 3 indiv. or 1 oz
eggs 1
vienna sausage.. 2
wiener... 1
cold cuts .... 1 oz

Note: Additional foods that can be used like meat exchanges (*i.e.*, cheeses) can be found in the Dairy Group Exchange List. Bacon, although a meat, is listed under the fats category.

2: FRUIT EXCHANGE LIST

One exchange contains approximately 10 grams of carbohydrate and 40 calories.

apple .... 1 sm
apple juice... ⅓ cup
    cider.. ⅓ cup
applesauce, unsweetened................................. ½ cup
apricots, fresh.. 2 med
apricots, dried... 4 halves
banana... ½ sm
berries:
    blackberries... ½ cup
    blueberries.. ½ cup

cranberries .... ½ cup
raspberries .... ½ cup
strawberries .... ¾ cup
cherries .... 10 lge
dates 2
figs, fresh 1
figs, dried 1
grapefruit .... ½ cup
grapefruit juice .... ½ cup
grapes 12
grape juice .... ¼ cup
lemon, raw 2
lemon juice... ½ cup
mango .... ½ sm
melons:
    cantaloupe .... ¼ sm
    honeydew .... ⅛ med
    watermelon.. 1 cup
nectarine.. 1 sm
orange .... 1 sm
orange juice .... ½ cup
papaya.. ¾ cup
peach .... 1 med
    canned, syrup .... 3 tbsp
    canned, water-packed .... ½ cup
pear .... 1 sm
    canned, syrup .... 3 tbsp
persimmon, native.. 1 med
pineapple, raw, cubed, canned, syrup, crushed,
    chunks... 3 tbsp
    juice... ⅓ cup
plums.. 2 med
    canned, syrup (with pits) .... 3 tbsp
prunes .... 2 med
prune juice .... ¼ cup
raisins .... 2 tbsp
tangerine.. 1 med

3: BREAD EXCHANGE LIST

One exchange of bread contains approximately 13 grams of carbohydrate, 2 grams of protein, 1 gram of fat, 70 calories.

breads:
white	1 sl
French	1 sl
Italian	1 sl
whole wheat	1 sl
rye	1 sl
pumpernickel	1 sl
raisin	1 sl
bagel	½
biscuit roll (2″ diam)	1
English muffin	½
plain roll	1 sm
frankfurter roll	½
hamburger bun	½
dried breadcrumbs	3 tbsp
tortilla, 6″	1
matzoh (6″ diam)	1
corn bread (1.5″ cube)	1
corn muffin	1
muffin, plain	1 sm

cereals:
bran flakes	½ cup
other ready-to-eat cereal, unsweetened	¾ cup
puffed cereal, unfrosted	1 cup
cereal, cooked	½ cup
grits, cooked	½ cup
rice or barley, cooked	½ cup
pasta, cooked, without sauce	
spaghetti	½ cup
noodles	½ cup
macaroni	½ cup

popcorn, popped, plain .... 3 cups
   with oil .... 2 cups
cornmeal, dry .... 2 tbsp
flour, all-purpose enriched .... 2½ tbsp
   self-rising .... 2½ tbsp
wheat germ .... 1 tbsp
pancake (5½" diam) 1
waffle (5½" diam) 1
crackers:
   arrowroot 3
   graham (2½" sq) 2
   oyster 20
   variety .... 5 sm
   pretzels (3" long × ⅛" diam) 25
   rye wafers (2" × 3½") 3
   saltines 6
   soda (2½" sq) 4
   round butter type 5

Veggie-Breads

Some vegetables and vegetable-related products are also included under the Bread Exchange List. There's a very sensible reason for this. These veggies have an almost identical nutritional profile, in the balance of carbohydrate and protein that they contain, to their cousins in the bread category. The only difference is that they contain little or no fat (except where specified).

When you get to the menus section, you will see that they are identified as bread exchanges on the menu lists.

parsnips .... ⅔ cup
corn .... ½ cup
   on the cob .... 1 med ear
potatoes, sweet, or yams, cooked .... ¼ cup
   white, baked (2" diam) 1
   white, boiled (2" diam) 1

white, mashed with milk .... ½ cup
french fries .... 8 med
chips .... 10 lg
pumpkin .... 1 cup
squash, winter (acorn or butternut).................... ½ cup

Cakes, Cookies, and Pies

For those of you with a sweet tooth, don't despair; cakes, cookies, and pies can be a delightful addition to your diet. Unlike other dietary regimens, the Pain-Free Diet welcomes these desserts because they are high in carbohydrate content. But there is a price to pay with the additional fats and calories. Again, for this reason, we have included a complete nutritional profile so you can make your individual choices to blend them in with your daily menus.

| | ---------- grams---------- | | | |
	Prot	Fat	Carb	Cals
cakes				
coffee (⅙ of round cake)	5	7	38	230
yellow (⅙ of round cake)	3	8	45	250
pound (1 sl)	2	10	16	160
danish, plain (4.5″ diam)	5	15	30	175
doughnut, plain	1	5	13	100
doughnut, glazed	3	11	22	205
cookies				
brownie with nuts	1	6	10	95
chocolate chip (4)	3	8	38	235
fig bar (4)	2	3	42	200
oatmeal, with raisins (4)	3	8	38	235
pies (9″ diam); 1 portion = ⅐ of pie				
banana cream, custard	7	13	35	285
fruit (apple, blueberry, cherry, peach)	3	15	50	345

| | --------- *grams* ---------- | | | |
	Prot	Fat	Carb	Cals
lemon meringue	4	12	45	305
pecan	6	27	61	495
pumpkin	5	15	32	275

Beans and Legumes

A third section of veggie-breads, the legumes and beans, is included with a breakdown of their nutritional content. These tend not to fit exactly into the bread profile, while still retaining most of the bread character. You can make your own adjustments as desired by following their exact protein/carbohydrate/fat contents.

One exchange contains 7 grams of protein, .5 gram of fat, 20 grams of carbohydrate. Each yields 110 calories (notably more than the initial bread exchanges).

beans, dry, cooked .... ½ cup
lima beans .... ½ cup
lentils, cooked .... ½ cup
blackeye peas, dry, cooked .... ½ cup
green peas, canned, frozen .... ¾ cup
split peas, dry, cooked .... ½ cup

4: VEGETABLES EXCHANGE LIST

The following raw vegetables are *unrestricted*—that is, they can be used in any quantities as desired:

chicory	lettuce
Chinese cabbage	parsley
endive	radishes
escarole	watercress

One exchange of the following vegetables contains approximately 2 grams of protein, 5 grams of carbohydrate, 0 grams of fat, 25 calories.

asparagus	1 cup
bean sprouts, raw	½ cup
beets	½ cup
broccoli	½ cup
brussels sprouts	½ cup
cabbage	1 cup
carrots	½ cup
cauliflower	1 cup
celery	1 cup
cucumber	6 sl
eggplant	½ cup
greens:	
beets	1 cup
chard	½ cup
collard	½ cup
dandelion	1 cup
kale	1 cup
mustard	1 cup
spinach, raw	1 cup
turnip	1 cup
mushrooms, raw	1 cup
okra, cooked	10 pods
onions, raw	1 cup
peppers, green	1 cup
sauerkraut	½ cup
squash, summer	1 cup
string beans, green or yellow	1 cup
tomato, or tomato juice	½ cup
turnip	1 cup
vegetable juice cocktail	½ cup
zucchini	½ cup

Note: If you didn't find certain vegetables, like potatoes and yams, for example, this is because their unique nutritional makeup places them in the Bread Exchange List section.

5: DAIRY GROUP EXCHANGE LIST

One exchange of fat-free milk contains approximately 8 grams of protein, 12 grams of carbohydrate, 80 calories.

skim or nonfat... 1 cup
powdered (before adding liquid)......................... ⅓ cup
yogurt (made from skim milk)............................ 1 cup
buttermilk (made from skim milk)...................... 1 cup
canned, evaporated skim milk.......................... ½ cup
whole milk (in addition to protein and carbohydrate,
   whole milk contains fat) 3.3% butter fat
   (8 gm fat, 150 cal)....................................... 1 cup
2% butter fat (5 gm fat, 125 cal) .... 1 cup
1% butter fat (3 gm fat, 105 cal) .... 1 cup
buttermilk (2 gm fat, 100 cal)........................... 1 cup

Dairy Products That May Be Used as Meat-Exchange Alternatives

Because some dairy products (especially cheeses) are high in protein they may be used as meat-exchange alternatives. But beware: They are also loaded with fat, and some can pack a powerful caloric punch.

For example, portions of cheeses may vary from as little as 90 calories per suggested serving with 7 grams of fat, to a whopping 428 calories with a heavy 32 grams of fat!

Many people live under the misconception that they are getting only a quick protein boost when they eat cheese—but as you will see, depending on the variety of cheese, you may be paying a heavy fat penalty.

Because of the vast nutritional variety the following table gives a very precise nutritional breakdown of these dairy products so you can accurately judge for yourself when you use them, either individually or as a meat-exchange alternative.

Do not forget to balance out your daily menu plan by eliminating other (mainly fat-content) foods to fit the required protein/carbohydrate/fat profile when picking from the following list.

		---------- *grams* ----------			
		Prot	Fat	Carb	Cals
cheeses (natural)					
blue	1 oz	6	8	1	100
Camembert	1 wedge	8	9	—	115
cheddar	1 oz	7	9	—	115
cottage					
curd	1 cup	27	9	6	225
cream					
(2% fat)	1 cup	31	4	8	205
(1% fat)	1 cup	28	2	6	165
cream	1 oz	2	10	1	100
mozzarella					
whole milk	1 oz	6	7	1	90
part skim	1 oz	8	5	1	80
provolone	1 oz	7	8	1	100
ricotta					
whole milk	1 cup	28	32	7	428
part skim	1 cup	28	19	13	340
Swiss	1 oz	8	8	1	105
cheeses (processed)					
American	1 oz	6	9	—	105
Swiss	1 oz	7	7	1	95
sour cream	1 tbsp	—	3	1	25
yogurt, lowfat milk					
plain	8 oz	12	4	16	145
fruit	8 oz	10	3	42	230
pudding					
regular	1 cup	9	8	59	320
ice cream					
11% fat	1 cup	5	14	32	270
custard	1 cup	7	23	38	375

6: FATS EXCHANGE LIST

One exchange contains approximately 4 grams fat and 35 calories.

margarine (stick or tub)	1 tsp
butter	1 tsp
lard	1 tsp
oils:	
corn	1 tsp
cottonseed	1 tsp
safflower	1 tsp
soy	1 tsp
sunflower	1 tsp
olive	1 tsp
peanut	1 tsp
cream:	
heavy	1 tbsp
sour	2 tbsp
light	2 tbsp
salad dressings (regular):	
blue cheese	1 tsp
French	1 tsp
Italian	1 tsp
Thousand Island	1 tsp
mayonnaise	1 tsp
salad dressings (lo-cal):	
blue cheese	2 tbsp
French	2 tbsp
Italian	2 tbsp
Thousand Island	2 tbsp
mayonnaise	2 tbsp
olives	5 small
bacon	1 slice

Nuts

Because there is a great variety of nuts with widely varying nutritional and caloric contents, consult the following handy table for a precise breakdown.

		--------- grams ----------			
		Prot	**Fat**	**Carb**	**Cals**
almonds	½ cup	12	35	12	400
Brazil	6–8 indiv	4	19	13	184
cashew	½ cup	12	32	20	400
hazelnut	½ cup	8	42	12	425
macadamia	6 indiv	2	12	2	110
peanuts	½ cup	18	35	14	420
pecans	½ cup	6	40	9	405
pistachio	30 indiv	3	8	3	90
pumpkin	½ cup	20	35	10	400
sunflower	½ cup	18	35	15	405
walnuts	½ cup	9	40	10	400
peanut butter (no sugar)	1 tbsp	4	8	3	95

ADDITIONAL HELPFUL FOODS, SWEETS, SNACKS, AND BEVERAGES

The following two tables include additional eats and drinks that you may want to include in your dietary plan. Individually (in moderation), they will not upset the balance of your protein/carbohydrate/fat intake to any significant degree.

But we have listed caloric contents for the serious calorie counter.

Sugars and Sweets

	Serving	Cals
caramels	1 oz	115
chocolate: milk,		
semisweet	1 oz	145
chocolate peanuts	1 oz	160
fudge	1 oz	115
gumdrops	1 oz	100
honey	1 tbsp	65
jams	1 tbsp	55
jellies	1 tbsp	50
syrups		
chocolate-flavored	2 tbsp	90
chocolate, fudge	2 tbsp	125
molasses	1 tbsp	50
blackstrap	1 tbsp	45
table blends	1 tbsp	60
sugars		
brown	1 tbsp	50
white	1 tbsp	45
powdered	1 tbsp	24

Beverages

NONALCOHOLIC

	Serving	Cals
Water		
carbonated	12 fl oz	0
carbonated sweet	12 fl oz	115
colas	12 fl oz	145
fruit sodas	12 fl oz	170

	Serving	Cals
Tom Collins mix	12 fl oz	170
ginger ale	12 fl oz	115
root beer	12 fl oz	150

ALCOHOLIC

	Serving	Cals
beer	12 fl oz	150
gin, rum, vodka, whisky		
80 proof	1.5 fl oz	95
86 proof	1.5 fl oz	105
90 proof	1.5 fl oz	110
100 proof	1.5 fl oz	120
wines		
table	3.5 fl oz	85
dessert	3.5 fl oz	140

SMART SNACKING

Smart snacking is simple if you select healthful snacks from the basic food groups anytime you feel you need a lift.

Fruits and Vegetables

A crunchy apple, a banana, a pear, a bunch of grapes, a crisp carrot, and celery or zucchini sticks are all easy snack choices and provide fiber, vitamins, and minerals.

Fruits such as oranges and grapefruits are particularly good. They have vitamin C, which you need daily. Tomatoes and green peppers are excellent sources of vitamins A and C.

Juices are also a good choice instead of a soft drink. And the next time you want to reach for a bag of chips or cookies, make yourself a salad instead.

Dairy Foods

Milk, cheese, and yogurt are instant snacks packed with calcium, riboflavin, protein, vitamins A and D, and phosphorus, but do remember that many have a high fat content. Try being creative and make your own energy drinks using milk, yogurt, and fruit flavorings.

Cereals and Breads

Grains, especially whole grains, provide B vitamins, minerals, protein, and fiber. Snack on a piece of toast or use breads as a base for making a delicious sandwich.

Alternatives

A leftover chicken leg or sardines can dress up a salad or make an exciting snack, especially when you're on the go. And do-ahead fillings, like tuna fish and ham or egg salad, not only keep well when refrigerated but are great for lunches or as in-between treats when piled on crackers. Warning: Do not make snacks the night before or in the morning for lunchtime if they cannot be refrigerated between times.

Note: Go easy on the snacks. Everyone should really minimize this habit rather then encourage it. Eat properly and don't get into the habit of snacking all the time. The snacks provided between meals in the higher calorie levels of the Pain-Free Diet should be quite sufficient.

8

THE TRYPTOPHAN KEY

Now we come to the real heart of the Pain-Free Diet—boosting your daily tryptophan potential.

In the previous chapters you have learned how to program your own personal diet and why you need the proper balanced diet, one with modest amounts of complete protein, higher proportions of carbohydrate, and lower fat intake. With this combination you are providing the optimum conditions to assist the transfer of tryptophan across the blood-brain barrier to increase your levels of brain serotonin.

For the individual who is already free of pain and wants to stay that way, the Pain-Free Diet will help to maintain this condition of good health. If a person is troubled by chronic intractable pain, then the most effective way to begin nutritional treatment is to assist the body by taking supplemental tryptophan in addition to that already present in the foods of the Pain-Free Diet. This is exactly what our patients did.

It is also essential to ensure that there are the desired levels of two other vitally important nutrients in the diet.

These are Vitamin B_6 (pyridoxine) and niacin, or niacinamide—the version of niacin that does not cause its unwanted hot or "flushing" effect. Vitamin B_6 activates an enzyme that is necessary to convert tryptophan to serotonin. With an insufficient intake of niacin, the body will in desperation transform tryptophan into niacin. To encourage the body to reserve tryptophan for its conversion to serotonin, supplemental niacin is included to minimize the body's need to make it from tryptophan. More about this shortly.

Fortunately, we need only small amounts of these two nutrients, and to assure that they are present we advise patients to take them in supplement form together with tryptophan at each meal.

HOW MUCH TRYPTOPHAN AND WHEN?

For those people who have chronic or intractable pain, the most effective way we have found to start a pain-reduction program is to suggest additional tryptophan at the very start and then gradually decrease the daily dosage as the body comes into nutritional balance and is able to make effective use of the tryptophan contained in the diet.

In our successful pain-reduction studies at Temple University, we began with an initial dose of 2,500 milligrams daily of tryptophan for the first week along with a properly balanced diet as already discussed. For most people the levels were later reduced to suit the subjects' own individual needs, and these lower levels were continued to help keep our patients pain-free.

Our studies showed that taking the additional tryptophan in one dose each day, even with a meal, will markedly decrease its effectiveness. To ensure the tryptophan is provided to the body in the amounts that can be easily utilized divide the 2,500 milligram dose into smaller doses and spread them throughout the day, preferably with each meal and the bedtime snack. Since the average capsule or tablet of tryptophan contains 500 mg, one way of spreading the intake would be to take 500 mg at breakfast, at lunch, and at dinner, plus 1,000 mg with a carbohydrate snack prior to retiring.

Fortunately, supplemental tryptophan is remarkably safe and free of adverse long-term side effects. Long-term studies in Britain, where tryptophan supplementation is used by physicians in a number of emotional and psychiatric disorders, have shown it to be free of any side effects no matter what the duration of prescription.

In the United States the FDA (Food and Drug Administration) considers L-tryptophan to be a Nutrient/Dietary Supplement, and it is contained in the government's Generally Recognized as Safe (GRAS) list. It is not classified as a drug.

B_6 (Pyridoxine) and Niacin

Vitamin B_6 is essential for both the utilization of proteins from the diet and because it is part of the enzyme system that functions in the conversion of tryptophan to serotonin. By providing the body with this vitamin at the same time the tryptophan is given, we help to ensure the optimum activity of this needed enzyme.

Niacin is another essential nutrient that the body must have at all times. Because of its importance, the body has evolved a method by which it can literally tear tryptophan apart like a tinker toy and make niacin from the pieces. As a matter of fact, studies in humans have shown that the amount of niacin the body gets from tryptophan is equal to about half the total amount of niacin (nicotinic acid) that the body needs every day; sixty milligrams of tryptophan is used by the body to make each milligram of niacin.

Since the average amount of niacin adults need each day ranges from 13 mg for women to 19 mg for men, this means that from 390 mg to 570 mg of tryptophan would be needed each day just to make niacin, unless the diet itself already contained niacin (or niacinamide).

To show how much dietary protein this would take, consider the following: With an average requirement of 3 mg of tryptophan per kilogram (2.2 pounds) of body weight per day, the average woman of 55 kg (about 120 lbs) needs 165 mg of tryptophan and the average man (about 73 kg, or 160 lbs) needs 219 mg.

The RDAs show us that the average amount of protein required daily ranges from 44 grams for women to 56 grams for men. Since we get about 11 mg of tryptophan from every gram (one twenty-eighth of an ounce) of protein we eat, fully one third of the total amount of protein needed each day (15 to 20 grams) is potentially used just to provide the tryptophan that the body allocates to make niacin!

It's easy to see, theoretically, that if anyone is deficient in niacin, not only will the body use one third of its daily protein to supply the tryptophan for conversion to niacin, but now there may be even more tryptophan (through protein) required to provide essential serotonin.

This action, which makes sure of sufficient levels of niacin, takes priority over most others involving tryptophan. The result is that the remaining amounts of tryptophan the body uses to make serotonin are also decreased. Eventually, this could cause a deficiency of tryptophan for serotonin production . . . with chronic pain as a possible result.

By taking niacin and B_6 along with the tryptophan we make certain that the body has (1) sufficient niacin, thus decreasing its dependence on using tryptophan to make niacin, and (2) enough of the B_6 that is important in helping the body convert tryptophan to serotonin.

The Best Ways to Get Your B₆ and Niacin

Taking separate B_6 and niacin supplements with daily tryptophan doses could solve the problem of maintaining adequate amounts of these vitamins. But there are now tryptophan capsules on the market, which contain B_6 and niacin together. We have favored this approach because it simplifies the whole operation. Prior to this, subjects on the Pain-Free Diet were told to be very careful to see that they were getting at least the recommended daily levels of B_6 and niacin: at least ten milligrams of B_6 and twenty to twenty-five milligrams of niacin (or niacinamide) each day.

The following products offer a balanced combination of L-tryptophan with either B_6, niacin, or both, and in some cases additional vitamins.

Trypto-Vite*(Patent Pending)

Manufacturer:
Commonwealth Medical Corporation of American
(The Preventive Medical Company)
751 N. 7th St.
Allentown, PA 18102

Each capsule contains:
L-tryptophan 250 mg
niacinamide 25 mg
B_6 25 mg
Fructose 250 mg

*Available mail order/selected retail outlets.

L-Tryptophan Plus*

Manufacturer:
Twin Laboratories, Inc.
2120 Smithtown Ave.
Ronkonkoma, NY 11779

Each capsule contains:
L-tryptophan 500 mg
B_6 10 mg
niacinamide 25 mg
vitamin C 100 mg

*Available in good health food stores.

L-Tryptophan with Niacinamide, B_6, and Vitamin C*

Supplier:
Dajean Gerontological Laboratories
P.O. Box 314
Lake Grove, NY 11755

Two capsules contain:
L-tryptophan 500 mg
B_6 10 mg
niacinamide 25 mg
vitamin C 100 mg

*Available by mail order only. Information book also available by mail.

Tryptophan P.R.N.* Nutri-Cology (brand)

Supplier:
Allergy Research Group
247 Eastend Way
Pleasant Hill, CA 94523

Each dosage contains:
L-tryptophan 350 mg

B_6 25 mg
niacinamide 50 mg

Available by mail order only.

Trypto-Vates*

Supplier:
Alacer Corp.
Buena Park, CA 90622

Each dosage contains:
L-tryptophan 500 mg
B_1 25 mg
B_2 25 mg
B_6 25 mg
biotin 100 mcg
vitamin C 50 mg

Does not contain niacin. Available in health food stores.

An Alternate Approach

Another option is to purchase tryptophan supplies separately and use a one-a-day, time-release multivitamin preparation that contains the required daily levels of B_6 and niacin. There's a sound reason for doing this. In such products the vitamins and minerals are formulated so that, after the tablets are swallowed, they dissolve slowly in the intestinal tract. This slow release of the nutrients occurs at a rate that enables the body to utilize them to their best advantage.

After most vitamin and mineral preparations are taken —in the morning with breakfast, for example—the tablet or capsule dissolves quickly in the stomach or small intestine. All of the vitamins and minerals that are released are absorbed at once.

Since the body cannot utilize all of these nutrients at the time they are made available, the body takes what it needs and gets rid of the rest. So, during the remainder of the twenty-four-hour period the nutrients that have been gotten rid of are now no longer available to the body when it needs them. This is the major reason it's important to use every meal—to spread out the supply of nutrients during the day and make them available to our body at a rate at which they can be best utilized.

A WORD ABOUT TRYPTOPHAN SUPPLIES

Tryptophan is available in a variety of dose sizes in most pharmacies and health food stores. During the development of the Pain-Free Diet, the 500 mg strength was found to be the most convenient. 1,000 mg (1 gm) tablets can also be easily utilized by breaking them in half to provide each 500 mg dose.

The following are easy-to-refer-to dos and don'ts when purchasing tryptophan supplies.

- Make sure the tryptophan supply is clearly labeled "L-tryptophan." Do not buy anything else.
- Do not purchase anything that says simply "tryptophan" or has a name that sounds similar to tryptophan: *i.e.*, Tryptofan, Triptophan, Triptofan, etc.
- Avoid tryptophan products that advertise themselves as natural. Consumers find they may well be paying extra for something that is essentially the same end product; only the manufacturing process is likely to be different.
- Always check the content part of the label very carefully for both individual tablet dosage and any other supplements or fillers that may be in the product.

GETTING STARTED ON AND FOLLOWING THE PROGRAM

Here is the timetable for tryptophan supplementation of the Pain-Free Diet, which was used successfully by our patients with intractable pain.

The goals are twofold: to provide pain relief as quickly as possible, and to find the simplest and least expensive maintenance program for each person to help stay pain-free.

To accomplish these goals, supplementation is begun with relatively high levels of tryptophan and the amounts are then slowly decreased to each individual's best maintenance level.

Initially, 500 mg doses of tryptophan are taken with each snack or meal, and later as the daily intake of tryptophan decreases the doses can be rearranged to suit individual preferences and needs. More about this after the schedule.

FIRST 5 DAYS: 500 mg of tryptophan with breakfast, at midmorning, lunch, dinner, and with the late-night snack. This makes a daily total of 2.5 gm taken together with B_6 and niacin.

6–14 DAYS: If the pain has moderated sufficiently, the tapering-off process may now begin. The supplements now consist of 500 mg of tryptophan with breakfast, lunch, dinner, and late-night snack. A total of 2 gm a day together with the recommended B_6 and niacin.

15–21 DAYS: 500 mg of tryptophan with lunch, dinner, and late-night snack. A total of 1,500 mg a day together with the B_6 and niacin.

22 DAYS AND AFTER: 500 mg of tryptophan at lunch and with your late-night snack. A total of 1,000 mg (1 gm) a day together with the B_6 and niacin.

INDIVIDUAL NEEDS

The perception of pain varies from person to person and even from moment to moment. Our metabolic and nutritional needs are also unique from person to person. This is why we have preferred to start the tryptophan regimen at a clinically increased level and bring it down so that individuals can recognize which level is most beneficial to their own needs.

We found that what pain subjects should expect to feel in the first few days is a very definite reduction of pain. Even in the following days and weeks, as the tryptophan intake is reduced, this beneficial effect continues. But if the tryptophan drops too low, pain might start increasing again; at this time patients are taught to recognize that they have gone below their individual tryptophan needs, so they simply step up their existing daily dosage by 500 milligrams.

One individual may find that for the most effective pain reduction, two grams of tryptophan are required, while another person may find one gram sufficient. It's all a matter of discovering your own appropriate tryptophan balance.

SLEEP PROBLEMS?

Once they have found their ideal tryptophan supplement levels, some people who suffer from insomnia or sleep disturbances prefer to take the largest dose of their daily tryptophan last thing at night. There is nothing wrong with this, as tryptophan plays a key role in the quality of sleep and its onset.

This approach is highly recommended (and, in fact, has been used for years by many psychiatrists) whenever sleep difficulties are a problem, and it does nothing to detract from the overall pain-free potential. The simple rule is to make sure that the late-night snack is rich in carbohydrate (refer to Chapter 9 for late-night snacks) and the tryptophan is taken with it an hour or thirty minutes before retiring.

CONSULT WITH YOUR FAMILY PHYSICIAN

We cannot stress the importance of visiting a physician before starting any new nutritional program or diet, and this includes the Pain-Free Diet.

First, your pain may be a signal of some disease process that should be diagnosed and treated to remove the specific cause of the pain. But even when this turns out not to be the case, there are two additional benefits. A regular checkup from your doctor at the start of a diet will ascertain whether there is anything in your physical condition that could be detrimental to utilizing the Pain-Free Diet successfully, and it will allow your physician to record your progress on the diet accurately.

Do not hesitate to take this book along with you to the physician's office so that your medical professional can acquaint himself with the program.

DO NOT SELF-MEDICATE!

It is essential that you do not discontinue or reduce any medications that have been prescribed for you by a physician. It can be dangerous to take the administration of prescription drugs into your own hands.

If you are on painkilling, or anti-inflammatory, drugs, visit with your physician and tell him about your intentions to start the Pain-Free nutritional program—especially if you intend to utilize tryptophan-boosting supplements. Seek his advice and have a frank discussion about the pros and cons of your proposed new dietary regimen. Follow your physician's instructions to the letter.

In most cases a physician will respect your wishes to follow a nutritionally sound new lifestyle to combat your pain problems, but he may want to observe your progress over a period of time before making a decision to reduce or eliminate present medications.

While developing the Pain-Free Diet we have observed patients who have been at their wits' end with intractable pain (even to the point of contemplating suicide) suddenly find genuine relief for the first time in their lives. They were then able to follow reduced medication levels, and some could eventually eliminate them altogether.

PREGNANT WOMEN: A CAUTION!

Although a deficiency of tryptophan has been found in women suffering from depression shortly after giving birth, new research in animals may indicate that the presence of high serotonin levels during pregnancy could have adverse effects on the unborn child.

Studies conducted at Louisiana State University are very tentative, and this potential problem has been observed only in animal models. But, because our primary concern is for good health and safety, we must stress that it may not be advisable for a childbearing female to take dietary tryptophan supplements.

The research program in the department of zoology and physiology at Louisiana State found that the litter size and birthweights of golden hamsters were both significantly reduced in direct proportion to the increased amounts of supplemental dietary tryptophan fed to them during pregnancy.

For example, a normal tryptophan level (1 percent of the protein intake), combined with a medium protein diet, produced the highest litter size of almost ten offspring with weights around 2.5 grams. A group fed a massive 8 percent of tryptophan with a medium protein intake produced litters of less than four offspring with average weights of just over 1.5 grams.

We are not aware of any research that as yet confirms this same effect in humans.

SEROTONIN AND THE ASTHMATIC

A specific anomaly concerning serotonin has been noted among sufferers of chronic asthma. European studies have shown that bronchial constriction may be promoted by the action of serotonin.

In view of this finding, we strongly suggest that anyone with a diagnosed asthmatic condition consult with his or her physician before making any dietary changes that might affect the body's natural serotonin balance.

9

MENUS FOR EVERY
WEIGHT GOAL

In this chapter you will find a variety of menus created from the exchange lists in Chapter 7.

The value of working with the exchange-list system is that you can concoct any menu to fit the occasion, whether you want a quick lunchtime snack or are preparing a special anniversary dinner. The series of sample menus we present in this chapter can be used as they are, or you can mix and match the menus and create new daily plans.

Don't forget all the gourmet tricks you might ordinarily use in your own kitchen: things like spices and flavorings, special ways of preparing and cooking. In fact, as long as you are not altering the balance of the ingredients, almost anything goes. You can use your own imagination, and at the end of this chapter we've also given you handy tips for enhancing certain foods.

The sample menus have been constructed on four specific calorie levels: 1,000, 1,500, 2,000, and 3,000.

You simply pick the calorie level you want to follow for your desired goal. You will have worked out your ideal weight and dietary requirements from the previous chapters on learning to eat smart and discovering what's wrong with the American diet.

If you want a safe but sensibly quick weight-loss diet, you may want to consider the 1,000-calorie regimen—but we suggest you do not continue this for more than three weeks at any given time. You can change to a higher calorie level for two weeks and then come back to the 1,000-calorie level.

The other diet levels have increasing calorie totals, but they still stick to the required balance of protein, carbohydrate, and fat.

You will also notice that the 1,000-calorie diet gives a very specific breakdown of how much of the different nutrients are contained in each meal, and how many calories they provide. This illustrates what happens when you pick your food choices from the exchange lists. In the higher calorie levels we have simplified this to indicate just the exchange-list amounts.

To select which calorie level is right for you, consider that the 1,000 level should be viewed as a weight-loss program only, 1,500 as a weight-loss and maintenance regimen, and 2,000–3,000 as normal dietary levels, and also for increasing weight for those underweight individuals who may need it.

Last, don't be afraid to experiment with the meal combinations in any order; just because it's breakfast doesn't mean you can't have a hot roast-beef sandwich or a cup of ice cream. But if you do skip a meal, or any part of a meal, do remember to account for it in the menu for the total day. Don't forget it's the overall daily totals that count!

A SPECIAL VITAMIN AND MINERAL NOTE ON THE 1,000-CALORIE LEVEL

There is growing concern today among health professionals about the inability of a 1,000-calorie-a-day diet to supply all the essential vitamins and minerals through its nutritional content.

Even though you will be getting excellent guidance regarding the selection of foods containing the proper proportion of protein, carbohydrate, and fat, the chances are that they might be deficient when it comes to a daily total for the RDAs. This is so unpredictable at a low level of caloric intake because many foods lose some of their vitamin and mineral contents through shelf-life and processing—and this can be a crucial factor.

It's not always easy to guarantee that the California-grown head of lettuce you buy in Boston will have the same vitamin and mineral quantity and quality as the one purchased in Los Angeles—just a day or two in packaging and shipping can dramatically rob some produce of its nutritional qualities.

It is for this reason that we strongly suggest you accompany the 1,000-calorie-a-day levels with a one-a-day multivitamin/mineral supplement that contains all the required RDAs. If you are not sure exactly how much the RDAs are, check the tables in Chapter 4 and compare them with the listings on the package containing the supplement you choose.

We also emphasize that slow (or time-release) multivitamins are preferable over regular one-a-day products, which may lose much of their potential by being absorbed by the body too quickly. With speedy absorption the body can end up excreting much of the value of the nutrients because it has no call for them at that particular time of the day—although it might well need some of these important vitamins and minerals later in the twenty-four-hour cycle. Obviously, slow release will give a more controlled and comprehensive coverage.

A FURTHER WORD ABOUT TRYPTOPHAN SUPPLEMENTS

With the 3,000-calorie diet level you will see that it is broken down into 3 main daily meals and three snacks. This has made taking tryptophan supplements easy when subjects have started on the 2.5-gram-a-day level, taking each one of five daily supplements with the meals, and with two of the snacks. As daily tryptophan levels are reduced, supplements are then taken in the morning, at noon, and at bedtime.

Starting on one of the other dietary levels (*i.e.*, 1,000, 1,500, 2,000) you will notice that these daily menus have only three main meals and one bedtime snack. When subjects begin with five 500 mg doses of tryptophan a day, they take one dose midmorning with either a fruit or carbohydrate snack and then eliminate this (the snack food) from one of the three daily meal plans. Or, alternatively, the same is done in midafternoon, and again the food used as a snack is eliminated. For example, on the first Monday of the 1,500 level one might want to have a ½ cup pineapple juice from breakfast as a midmorning snack, or take two slices of bread from lunchtime to make a midafternoon toast snack.

1,000 CALORIES

MONDAY

| | ---------grams---------- | | | |
	Prot	Fat	Carb	Cals
Breakfast				
½ cup orange juice	—	—	10	40
½ sm banana	—	—	10	40
¾ cup dry cereal	2	1	13	70
1 cup skim milk	8	—	12	85
Lunch				
ham and cheese open sandwich				
1 sl whole wheat bread	2	1	13	70
1½ oz boiled ham	7.5	7.5	—	100
mustard, lettuce, carrot sticks,				
celery sticks	2	—	5	25
1 sm orange	—	—	10	40
1 cup skim milk	8	—	12	85
Dinner				
2 oz broiled fish	14	4	—	110
1 tsp cooking oil	—	5	—	45
½ cup tossed salad	2	—	5	25
½ cup cooked cauliflower	2	—	5	25
½ cup cubed pineapple	—	—	10	40
½ cup skim milk	4	—	6	40
Bedtime snack				
1 cup unsweetened applesauce	—	—	20	80
6 round thin crackers	2	—	15	70
Totals	53.5	18.5	146	990

TUESDAY

| | ---------- *grams* ---------- | | | |
	Prot	Fat	Carb	Cals
Breakfast				
½ cup orange juice	—	—	10	40
½ cup oatmeal	2	1	13	70
½ cup skim milk	4	—	6	40
1 tsp raisins	—	—	5	20
Lunch				
chef salad				
1 cup raw vegetables	2	—	5	25
1 sm tomato, cut up	2	—	5	25
1 oz (total) ham, cheese, chicken	7	2	—	55
1 tsp lo-cal dressing	—	.5	.5	5
3 rye wafers	2	1	13	70
½ cup skim milk	4	—	6	40
1 apple	—	—	10	40
Dinner				
¾ cup spaghetti with meatballs in				
tomato sauce	14	9	29	247
1 cup mixed salad	2	—	5	25
1 slice toasted garlic bread	2	1	13	70
1 tsp butter	—	5	—	45
½ cup skim milk	4	—	6	40
18 grapes	—	—	15	60
Bedtime snack				
¼ honeydew melon	—	—	20	80
Totals	45	19.5	161.5	997

WEDNESDAY

	Prot	*grams* Fat	Carb	Cals

Breakfast

	Prot	Fat	Carb	Cals
½ cup grapefruit juice	—	—	10	40
½ toasted bagel	2	1	13	70
2 tsp peanut butter	2	6	2	64
½ cup skim milk	4	—	6	40

Lunch

	Prot	Fat	Carb	Cals
1 cup vegetable soup	2	2	13	80
chicken sandwich				
2 sl whole wheat bread	4	2	26	140
1 oz sliced chicken	7	2	—	55
lettuce (as desired)				
1 sl tomato				
2 tsp lo-cal dressing	—	1	1	10
½ cup skim milk	4	—	6	40
1 cup melon balls	—	—	10	40

Dinner

	Prot	Fat	Carb	Cals
½ cup tomato juice	—	—	5	20
2 oz roast beef	14	4	—	110
½ cup cooked rice	2	—	13	70
¼ cup cooked zucchini	1	—	2.5	13
½ cup skim milk	4	—	6	40
2 cooked pear halves (water-packed)	—	—	10	40

Bedtime snack

	Prot	Fat	Carb	Cals
⅓ cup apple juice	—	—	10	40
1 sl raisin bread	2	1	13	65
Totals	48	19	146.5	977

THURSDAY

	Prot	Fat	Carb	Cals
	---------grams----------			

Breakfast

	Prot	Fat	Carb	Cals
½ grapefruit	—	—	10	40
1 shredded-wheat biscuit	2	1	20	90
1 cup skim milk	8	—	12	85

Lunch

	Prot	Fat	Carb	Cals
1 egg, any style	6	6	—	80
¼ cup sliced cucumber	1	—	2.5	13
¼ cup cherry tomatoes	1	—	2.5	13
2 tsp lo-cal dressing	—	1	1	10
3 whole wheat wafers	2	1	13	70
½ cup skim milk	4	—	6	40
1 med tangerine	—	—	10	40

Dinner

	Prot	Fat	Carb	Cals
beef kabob				
2 oz beef chunks	14	4	—	110
½ cup zucchini	2	—	5	25
¼ cup mushrooms	1	—	2.5	13
½ cup cherry tomatoes	2	—	5	25
½ cup cooked rice	2	—	13	70
1 tsp butter	—	4	—	35
½ cup skim milk	4	—	6	40
2 med plums	—	—	10	40

Bedtime snack

	Prot	Fat	Carb	Cals
1 cup cubed pineapple	—	—	20	80
3 graham crackers	2	1	13	70
Totals	51	18	151.5	989

FRIDAY

| | ---------grams---------- | | | |
	Prot	Fat	Carb	Cals
Breakfast				
½ cup grapefruit juice	—	—	10	40
1 cup plain yogurt	8	7	11	140
½ cup blueberries	—	—	10	40
Lunch				
grilled-cheese sandwich				
1 slice whole grain bread	2	1	13	70
1 oz cheddar cheese	7	9	—	115
¼ cup sliced mushrooms	1	—	2.5	13
2 sl tomato	1	—	2.5	13
1 tsp lo-cal mayonnaise	—	.5	.5	5
1 cup carrot and celery slices	2	—	5	25
½ cup skim milk	4	—	6	40
¾ cup strawberries	—	—	10	40
Dinner				
2 oz salmon (baked)	14	4	—	110
½ cup steamed cauliflower	2	—	5	25
½ cup baked winter squash	2	—	13	70
1 tsp butter	—	4	—	35
½ cup skim milk	4	—	6	40
½ cantaloupe	—	—	20	80
Bedtime snack				
½ grapefruit	—	—	10	40
1 tbsp honey on grapefruit	—	—	17	65
Totals	47	25.5	141.5	1,006

SATURDAY

	Prot	Fat	Carb	Cals
	---------grams----------			

Breakfast

	Prot	Fat	Carb	Cals
1 sm orange	—	—	10	40
1 poached egg	6	6	—	80
1 sl whole grain toast	2	1	13	70
1 tsp butter	—	4	—	35
½ cup skim milk	4	—	6	40

Lunch

turkey sandwich				
1 oz lean meat	7	2	—	55
2 sl whole grain bread	4	2	26	140
2 tsp mayonnaise	—	5	.5	50
1 sl tomato	.5	—	1.25	6.5
½ cup skim milk	4	—	6	40
2 med plums	—	—	10	40

Dinner

2 oz baked chicken (without skin)	14	4	—	110
½ cup mixed vegetable salad	2	—	5	25
1 tbsp lo-cal dressing	—	1	1	15
¼ cup cooked beets	1	—	7.5	35
1 dinner roll	2	1	13	70
½ cup skim milk	4	—	6	40
½ cup raspberries	—	—	10	40

Bedtime snack

1 med banana	—	—	26	100
Totals	50.5	26	141.25	1,031.5

SUNDAY

| | --------- grams ---------- | | | |
	Prot	**Fat**	**Carb**	**Cals**
Breakfast				
½ cup orange juice	—	—	10	40
½ cup Cream of Wheat	2	1	13	70
1 tsp butter	—	4	—	35
1 cup skim milk	8	—	12	85
Lunch				
1 cup minestrone soup	5	3	14	105
3 rye wafers	2	1	13	70
1 tsp butter	—	4	—	35
½ cup skim milk	4	—	6	40
1 sm orange	—	—	10	40
Dinner				
¼ cup cooked crab meat	7	2	—	55
1 sm baked potato	2	—	13	70
1 tbsp plain yogurt	.5	.4	.7	10
½ cup steamed asparagus	2	—	5	25
1 sl whole wheat bread	2	1	13	70
24 grapes	—	—	20	80
½ cup skim milk	4	—	6	40
Bedtime snack				
½ cup cranberry sauce	—	—	20	80
3 rye wafers	2	1	13	70
Totals	40.5	17.4	168.7	1,020

MONDAY

	Prot	Fat	Carb	Cals
		grams		

Breakfast

	Prot	Fat	Carb	Cals
½ cup grapefruit juice	—	—	10	40
1 boiled egg	6	6	—	80
1 sl whole grain bread	2	1	13	70
1 tsp butter	—	4	—	35
½ cup skim milk	4	—	6	40

Lunch

tuna sandwich

	Prot	Fat	Carb	Cals
¼ cup water-packed tuna	7	2	—	55
2 tbsp lo-cal mayonnaise	—	1	1	20
2 sl whole wheat bread	4	2	26	140
lettuce (as desired)				
½ cup skim milk	4	—	6	40
½ cup raspberries	—	—	10	40

Dinner

	Prot	Fat	Carb	Cals
2 oz sliced turkey	14	4	—	110
1 cup cauliflower topped with 1				
sl melted American cheese	6	9	—	105
1 cup watermelon	—	—	10	40

Bedtime snack

	Prot	Fat	Carb	Cals
1 cup applesauce	—	—	20	80
6 round crackers	2	1	13	70
Totals	**49**	**30**	**115**	**965**

TUESDAY

	Prot	Fat	Carb	Cals
	---------grams----------			

Breakfast

	Prot	Fat	Carb	Cals
½ cup orange juice	—	—	10	40
1 cup puffed wheat	2	1	13	70
½ cup skim milk	4	—	6	40
1 banana	—	—	20	80

Lunch

	Prot	Fat	Carb	Cals
¼ cup cottage cheese	7	2.5	1.5	60
3 whole wheat wafers	2	1	13	70
1 tsp butter	—	4	—	35
½ cup skim milk	4	—	6	40
1 cup fresh diced fruit	—	—	20	80

Dinner

	Prot	Fat	Carb	Cals
3 oz broiled beef patty	21	6	—	165
½ cup steamed asparagus	2	—	5	25
½ cup tossed green salad	2	—	5	25
½ cup skim milk	4	—	6	40
½ cantaloupe	—	—	20	80

Bedtime snack

	Prot	Fat	Carb	Cals
½ cup ice cream	2.5	7	16	135
Totals	50.5	21.5	141.5	985

WEDNESDAY

| | ---------*grams*---------- | | | |
	Prot	Fat	Carb	Cals
Breakfast				
½ cup orange juice	—	—	10	40
2 bran muffins	6	8	34	210
1 tsp butter	—	4	—	35
1 cup skim milk	8	—	12	85
Lunch				
mixed vegetable salad				
½ cup mixture of diced radishes, cucumbers, carrots, celery, red cabbage	2	—	5	25
1 tbsp lo-cal dressing	—	1.5	2	15
3 rye wafers	2	1	13	70
½ cup skim milk	4	—	6	40
½ cup grapefruit and orange sections	—	—	10	40
Dinner				
2 oz broiled liver	14	4	—	110
½ cup onions	1	—	7.5	30
1 tsp butter	—	4	—	35
½ cup cooked carrots	1	—	7.5	30
½ cup skim milk	4	—	6	40
1 sm pear	—	—	10	40
Bedtime snack				
1 sm baked potato	2	—	13	70
1 tbsp plain yogurt	.5	.5	1	9
⅔ cup apple juice	—	—	20	80
Totals	44.5	23	157	1,004

THURSDAY

| | --------- grams ---------- | | | |
	Prot	**Fat**	**Carb**	**Cals**
Breakfast				
½ cup orange juice	—	—	10	40
2 sl cornmeal brick (⅜″ × 1¾″ ×				
3¼″)	1.5	—	13	60
topped with 1 oz Swiss cheese	7	7	1	95
½ cup skim milk	4	—	6	40
Lunch				
macaroni/cheese casserole				
1 cup cooked whole wheat				
macaroni	4	2	26	140
1 oz cheddar cheese	7	9	—	115
½ cup skim milk	4	—	6	40
1 tangerine	—	—	10	40
Dinner				
2 oz filet of sole	14	4	—	110
1 sm baked potato	2	—	13	70
1 tsp butter	—	4	—	35
1 dinner roll	2	1	13	70
½ cup skim milk	4	—	6	40
2 fresh plums	—	—	10	40
Bedtime snack				
1 cup cubed fresh pineapple	—	—	20	80
Totals	49.5	27	134	1,015

FRIDAY

	Prot	Fat	Carb	Cals
	---------grams----------			

Breakfast

	Prot	Fat	Carb	Cals
½ sm grapefruit	—	—	10	40
½ cup cottage cheese	14	5	3	118
½ peach	—	—	10	40
½ cup skim milk	4	—	6	40

Lunch

	Prot	Fat	Carb	Cals
1 cup cream of tomato soup	7	7	23	175
2 breadsticks	2	1	13	70
1 cup vegetable salad	2	—	5	25
1 tbsp lo-cal salad dressing	—	1.5	2	15
1 cup skim milk	8	—	12	85
⅛ honeydew melon	—	—	10	40

Dinner
casserole

	Prot	Fat	Carb	Cals
½ cup rice	2	—	13	70
½ cup cooked lentils	7	—	20	110
¼ cup onions	1	—	7.5	30
1 tsp butter	—	4	—	35
½ cup skim milk	4	—	6	40
⅛ honeydew melon	—	—	10	40

Bedtime snack

	Prot	Fat	Carb	Cals
½ cup mixed fruit	—	—	10	40
Totals	51	18.5	160.5	1,013

SATURDAY

	--------- grams ----------			
	Prot	Fat	Carb	Cals
Breakfast				
½ cup grapefruit juice	—	—	10	40
½ cup bran flakes	2	1	13	70
½ sm banana	—	—	10	40
½ cup skim milk	4	—	6	40
Lunch				
chicken salad platter				
1 oz chicken	7	2	—	55
¼ cup diced celery and onions	1	—	5	21
½ cup tomato wedges	2	—	5	25
1 tbsp lo-cal dressing	—	1.5	2	15
6 small crackers	2	1	13	70
½ cup skim milk	4	—	6	40
1 peach	—	—	10	40
Dinner				
2 oz halibut steak	14	4	—	110
1 broiled tomato	2	—	5	25
1 biscuit	2	1	13	70
1 tsp butter	—	4	—	35
½ cup skim milk	4	—	6	40
1 cup watermelon balls	—	—	10	40
Bedtime snack				
1 cup cranberry sauce	—	—	42	165
3 graham crackers	2	1	13	70
Totals	46	15.5	169	1,011

SUNDAY

	grams			
	Prot	**Fat**	**Carb**	**Cals**
Breakfast				
½ cup orange juice	—	—	10	40
1 waffle	7	8	27	205
1 tbsp syrup	—	—	15	60
½ cup skim milk	4	—	6	40
Lunch				
peanut butter and celery sticks				
2 tbsp peanut butter	8	16	6	190
½ cup celery sticks	2	—	5	25
½ cup skim milk	4	—	6	40
1 sm orange	—	—	10	40
Dinner				
2 oz roast beef	14	4	—	110
¼ cup mashed potatoes	2	—	13	70
1 piece corn bread	2	1	13	70
1 tsp butter	—	4	—	35
½ cup skim milk	4	—	6	40
Bedtime snack				
½ cup mixed fresh fruit	—	—	10	40
Totals	47	33	127	1,005

1,500 CALORIES (approx)

A simple way to follow the 1,500 calorie regimen is to base it on this table:

Breakfast
2 fruit exchanges
1 meat exchange
2 bread exchanges
1 fat exchange
1 dairy exchange

Lunch
2 meat exchanges
2 bread exchanges
2 fat exchanges
1 vegetable exchange
2 fruit exchanges

Dinner
3 meat exchanges
2 bread exchanges
2 vegetable exchanges
vegetables (unrestricted) as desired
1 fruit exchange
1 fat exchange
½ dairy exchange

Bedtime snack
1 bread exchange
½ dairy exchange

MONDAY

Breakfast
½ cup pineapple juice (1 fruit exchange)
2 tbsp raisins (1 fruit)
1 egg, poached or boiled (1 meat)
1 sl toast (1 bread)
1 tsp butter or margarine (1 fat)
1 cup skim milk (1 dairy)

Lunch
½ cup tuna (1 fish)
2 sl bread (2 bread)
4 tsp mayonnaise (2 fat)
½ cup asparagus (1 vegetable)
2 sm apples (2 fruit)

Dinner
lettuce (as desired)
2 tsp Roquefort dressing (1 fat)
3 oz baked chicken (3 meat)
½ cup peas (1 starchy group B, considered a bread exchange)
½ cup mashed potatoes (1 starchy group B, considered a bread
    exchange)
½ mango (1 fruit)
½ cup skim milk (½ dairy)

Bedtime snack
4 graham crackers (2 bread)
½ cup skim milk (½ dairy)

TUESDAY

Breakfast
1 cup orange juice (2 fruit)
1 bagel (2 bread)
1 tsp butter (1 fat)
¼ cup cottage cheese (1 meat)
1 cup skim milk (1 dairy)

Lunch
1½ oz cold cuts (1 meat)
1 oz cheddar cheese (1 meat)
2 sl bread (2 bread)
2 tsp margarine or butter (2 fat)
½ cup sauerkraut (1 vegetable)
2 dates (1 fruit)

Dinner
5 scallops (1 meat)
6 sardines (2 meat)
1 English muffin (2 bread)
1 tsp butter (1 fat)
½ cup sautéd mushrooms (1 vegetable)
½ cup sautéd onions (1 vegetable)
watercress to garnish (as desired)
¾ cup mandarin oranges (1 fruit)
½ cup skim milk (½ dairy)

Bedtime snack
1½ cups popcorn (1 bread)
6 pretzels (1 bread)
½ cup skim milk (½ dairy)

WEDNESDAY

Breakfast
¼ cup wheat germ (1 bread)
1 cup grapefruit (2 fruit)
1 muffin (1 bread)
1 tsp butter or margarine (1 fat)
1 egg (1 meat)
1 cup skim milk (1 dairy)

Lunch
4 Vienna sausages (2 meat)
½ cup baked beans (2 bread)
½ cup tomato juice (1 vegetable)
¼ avocado (2 fat)
2 peaches (2 fruit)

Dinner
3 oz baked cheddar cheese in casserole dish (3 meat)
1 cup onions with cheese in casserole (2 vegetable)
1 tsp butter mixed in casserole (1 fat)
Chinese cabbage (as desired)
1 cup boiled potatoes (2 bread)
2 plums (1 fruit)
½ cup skim milk (½ dairy)

Bedtime snack
6 rye wafers (2 bread)
½ cup skim milk (½ dairy)

—————————————— **THURSDAY** ——————————————

Breakfast
1 English muffin (2 bread)
1 tsp butter or margarine (1 fat)
1 boiled egg (1 meat)
½ cup grape juice (2 fruit)
1 cup skim milk (1 dairy)

Lunch
½ cup salmon (2 meat)
2 sl bread (2 bread)
1 tsp margarine or butter (1 fat)
1 tsp mayonnaise (1 fat)
½ cup tomatoes (1 vegetable)
1 cup fruit cocktail (2 fruit)

Dinner
15 sm clams (3 meat)
1 tbsp light cream for sautéing clams (1 fat)
pepper to taste
2 tbsp flour to add to clams and cream (1 bread)
⅔ cup parsnips (1 bread)
1 cup cauliflower (2 vegetable)
radishes (as desired)
½ cup pineapple (1 fruit)
½ cup skim milk (½ dairy)

Bedtime snack
1 piece angel or sponge cake (2 bread)
½ cup skim milk (½ dairy)

FRIDAY

Breakfast
1½ cups cereal (2 bread)
4 tbsp raisins added to cereal (2 fruit)
¼ cup cottage cheese (1 meat)
6 sm nuts added to cereal (1 fat)
1 cup skim milk (1 dairy)

Lunch
1 omelet with 2 eggs (2 meat)
10 sm olives (2 fat)
1 cup rice or grits (2 bread)
1 cup brussels sprouts (2 vegetable)
1 med orange (2 fruit)

Dinner
3 oz lean hamburger (3 meat)
1 roll (1 bread)
½ cup spaghetti (1 bread)
½ cup carrots (1 vegetable)
½ cup bean sprouts (1 vegetable)
lettuce (as desired)
1 tbsp dressing (1 fat)
1 peach (1 fruit)
½ cup skim milk (½ dairy)

Bedtime snack
4 graham crackers (2 bread)
½ cup skim milk (½ dairy)

————————————— **SATURDAY** —————————————

Breakfast
1 sl crisp bacon (1 fat)
1 egg (1 meat)
2 muffins (2 bread)
2 fresh figs (2 fruit)
1 cup skim milk (1 dairy)

Lunch
2 oz lean pork chop (2 meat)
½ cup savory rice (1 bread)
½ cup peas (1 bread)
½ cup beets (1 vegetable)
lettuce (as desired)
2 tbsp Italian dressing (2 fat)
⅓ cup applesauce (1 fruit)
1 sm banana (1 fruit)

Dinner
3 oz lean steak (3 meat)
1 cup mashed potatoes (2 bread)
1 dinner roll (1 bread)
½ cup cabbage (1 vegetable)
½ cup green beans (1 vegetable)
endive (as desired)
1 tbsp cream cheese (1 fat)
1 lge tangerine (1 fruit)
½ cup skim milk (½ dairy)

Bedtime snack
6 saltines (1 bread)
½ cup skim milk (½ dairy)

SUNDAY

Breakfast
1 cup yogurt (1 dairy)
1 bagel (2 bread)
1 tsp butter (1 fat)
1 boiled egg (1 meat)
2 cups watermelon (2 fruit)

Lunch
3 fish sticks (1 bread, 2 meat)
1 sl bread (1 bread)
1 tsp butter or margarine (1 fat)
½ cup summer squash (1 vegetable)
1 med pear (2 fruit)

Dinner
10 med shrimp (3 meat)
lettuce (as desired)
½ cup raw mushrooms in salad (1 vegetable)
1 tbsp French dressing (1 fat)
1 tortilla (1 bread)
½ cup savory rice
2 lge plums (2 fruit)
½ cup skim milk (½ dairy)

Bedtime snack
½ cup wheat germ (2 bread)
½ cup skim milk (½ dairy)

MONDAY

Breakfast
1 cup orange juice (2 fruit)
3 med sardines (1 meat)
1 English muffin (2 bread)
1 tsp butter or margarine (1 fat)
1 cup skim milk (1 dairy)

Lunch
crab sandwich
2 sl whole wheat bread (2 bread)
½ cup crab (2 meat)
1 tsp butter or margarine (1 fat)
2 tsp lo-cal mayonnaise to mix with crab (1 fat)
1 cup cucumber slices (1 vegetable)
¼ honeydew melon (2 fruit)

Dinner
chef's salad
lettuce and ½ cup raw vegetables (1 vegetable)
1 med tomato cut up (1 vegetable)
1 oz shredded Swiss cheese (1 meat)
2 oz ham (2 meat)
1 tbsp low-cal dressing (1 fat)
1 cup spaghetti with sauce (2 bread)
1 dinner roll (1 bread)
1 cup skim milk (1 dairy)

Bedtime snack
¼ honeydew melon (1 fruit)
5 sm variety crackers (1 bread)

TUESDAY

Breakfast
1 cup grapefruit juice (2 fruit)
¾ cup dry cereal (1 bread)
1 sl white bread (1 bread)
1 egg (1 meat)
1 cup skim milk (1 dairy)

Lunch
1½ oz cold cuts (1 meat)
1 oz cheddar cheese (1 meat)
2 sl bread (2 bread)
½ cup carrot and celery sticks (1 vegetable)
2 sm apples (2 fruit)

Dinner
3 oz chicken legs and wings, fried (3 meat)
2½ tbsp flour with salt and pepper to coat chicken before frying
   (1 bread)
1 tsp oil or cooking fat (1 fat)
½ cup peas (1 bread)
½ cup broccoli (1 vegetable)
½ cup carrots (1 vegetable)
1 dinner roll (1 bread)
¾ cup strawberries (1 fruit)
½ cup skim milk (½ dairy)

Bedtime snack
2 graham crackers (1 bread)
½ cup skim milk (½ dairy)

WEDNESDAY

Breakfast
½ cup orange juice (1 fruit)
1 toasted bagel (2 bread)
1 egg (1 meat)
1 cup skim milk (1 dairy)

Lunch
salmon sandwich
½ cup salmon (2 meat)
2 sl whole wheat bread (2 bread)
½ cup celery sticks (1 vegetable)
½ cantaloupe (2 fruit)

Dinner
ham and cheese omelet
2 eggs (2 meat)
½ oz cheese (½ meat)
½ oz ham (½ meat)
1 cup mashed potatoes (2 bread)
½ cup zucchini (1 vegetable)
½ cup turnip (1 vegetable)
½ cup fruit cocktail (1 fruit)
½ cup skim milk (½ dairy)

Bedtime snack
20 lge potato chips (2 bread)
½ cup skim milk (½ dairy)

THURSDAY

Breakfast
1 sm grapefruit (2 fruit)
1 sl toast (1 bread)
1 tsp butter or margarine (1 fat)
1 cup skim milk (1 dairy)

Lunch
egg sandwich
2 hard-boiled eggs (2 meat)
2 sl white or brown bread (2 bread)
2 tsp mayonnaise (2 fat)
12 grapes (1 fruit)

Dinner
3 oz lean lamb chop (3 meat)
1 baked potato (1 bread)
parsley for garnish
1 cup bean sprouts (2 vegetable)
½ cup peas (1 bread)
lettuce (as desired)
2 tsp Roquefort dressing (1 fat)
1 apple (1 fruit)
½ cup skim milk (½ dairy)

Bedtime snack
4 graham crackers (2 bread)
½ cup skim milk (½ dairy)

FRIDAY

Breakfast
1 cup plain yogurt (1 dairy)
½ cup blueberries (1 fruit)
1 English muffin (2 bread)
1 tsp margarine or butter (1 fat)

Lunch
open-faced grilled-cheese sandwich
2 sl whole grain bread (2 bread)
2 oz cheddar cheese (2 meat)
¼ cup sliced mushrooms (½ vegetable)
2 sl tomato (½ vegetable)
⅔ cup apple juice (2 fruit)

Dinner
beef kabob
3 oz chunked beef (3 meat)
¼ cup zucchini (½ vegetable)
¼ cup tomatoes (½ vegetable)
¼ cup onions (½ vegetable)
¼ cup asparagus (½ vegetable)
½ cup peas (1 bread)
½ cup rice (1 bread)
½ cup pineapple (1 fruit)
½ cup skim milk (½ dairy)

Bedtime snack
½ cup ice cream, any flavor (1 bread, 2 fat)
2 graham crackers (1 bread)
½ cup skim milk (½ dairy)

SATURDAY

Breakfast
½ cup vegetable juice cocktail (1 vegetable)
1 med apple (2 fruit)
2 muffins (2 bread)
1 cup skim milk (1 dairy)

Lunch
shrimp sandwich
5 sm shrimp (3 meat)
2 sl white bread (2 bread)
2 tsp mayonnaise (2 fat)
1 cup orange juice (2 fruit)

Dinner
2 oz liver, sautéd (2 meat)
½ cup onions, sautéd (1 vegetable)
½ cup brussels sprouts (1 vegetable)
1 sl crisp bacon (1 fat)
1 cup mashed potatoes (2 bread)
1 oz grated cheddar cheese to mix with potatoes (1 meat)
10 lge cherries (1 fruit)
½ cup skim milk (½ dairy)

Bedtime snack
1 English muffin (2 bread)
1 tsp butter or margarine (1 fat)
½ cup skim milk (½ dairy)

SUNDAY

Breakfast
½ cup tomato juice (1 vegetable)
1 grapefruit (2 fruit)
1 poached egg (1 meat)
2 sl toast (2 bread)
1 tsp butter or margarine (1 fat)
1 cup skim milk (1 dairy)

Lunch
1 poached egg (1 meat)
1 oz ham (1 meat)
1 English muffin (2 bread)
1 tsp margarine or butter (1 fat)
½ cup asparagus (1 vegetable)
½ cup fruit cocktail (1 fruit)
½ cup orange juice (1 fruit)

Dinner
3 oz roast beef (3 meat)
2 baked potatoes (2 bread)
2 tbsp sour cream (2 fat)
½ cup cauliflower (1 vegetable)
½ cup carrots (1 vegetable)
2 med apricots (1 fruit)
½ cup skim milk (½ dairy)

Bedtime snack
12 pretzels (2 bread)
½ cup skim milk (½ dairy)

2,000 CALORIES (approx)

A simple way to follow the 2,000 calorie regimen is to base it on this table:

Breakfast
2 fruit exchanges
3 bread exchanges
2 fat exchanges
1 dairy exchange

Lunch
2 meat exchanges
3 bread exchanges
1 vegetable exchange
vegetables (unrestricted) as desired
2 fruit exchanges
1 fat exchange
1 dairy exchange

Dinner
3 meat exchanges
3 bread exchanges
2 vegetable exchanges
vegetables (unrestricted) as desired
1 fruit exchange
1 fat exchange
1 dairy exchange

Bedtime snack
3 bread exchanges
1 fruit exchange

MONDAY

Breakfast
1 English muffin (2 bread)
½ cup dry cereal (1 bread)
2 tsp butter or margarine (2 fat)
1 cup skim milk (1 dairy)
1 cup grapefruit juice (2 fruit)

Lunch
turkey sandwich
2 oz turkey (2 meat)
2 sl whole wheat bread (2 bread)
lettuce (as desired)
½ cup tomatoes sliced (1 vegetable)
2 tsp lo-cal mayonnaise (1 fat)
1 cup skim milk (1 dairy)
1 large pear (2 fruit)

Dinner
3 oz baked sole (3 meat)
1 cup peas (2 bread)
½ cup baked sweet potatoes (2 bread)
mixed greens salad (as desired)
2 tsp Roquefort dressing (1 fat)
12 grapes (1 fruit)
1 cup skim milk (1 dairy)

Bedtime snack
2 muffins (2 bread)
2 graham crackers (1 bread)
½ cup orange juice (1 fruit)

TUESDAY

Breakfast
1 cup grapefruit juice (2 fruit)
1 toasted bagel (2 bread)
1 tsp butter or margarine (1 fat)
1 cup skim milk (1 dairy)

Lunch
1½ oz cold cuts (1 meat)
1 oz sl Swiss cheese (1 meat)
4 sl whole wheat bread (4 bread)
2 tsp mayonnaise (2 fat)
½ cup asparagus (1 vegetable)
1 sm banana (2 fruit)
1 cup skim milk (1 dairy)

Dinner
5 scallops (1 meat)
6 sardines (2 meat)
1 cup savory rice (2 bread)
1 dinner roll (1 bread)
½ cup cooked cauliflower (1 vegetable)
½ cup brussels sprouts (1 vegetable)
1 tsp butter or margarine (1 fat)
1 small pear (1 fruit)
1 cup skim milk (1 dairy)

Bedtime snack
2 cups popcorn (2 bread)
6 saltines (1 bread)
½ cup pineapple juice (1 fruit)

WEDNESDAY

Breakfast
¼ cup wheat germ (1 bread)
1 toasted English muffin (2 bread)
2 tsp butter or margarine (2 fat)
1 cup flavored yogurt

Lunch
4 Vienna sausages (2 meat)
¾ cup baked beans (3 bread)
½ cup tomato juice (1 vegetable)
⅛ avocado (1 fat)
2 peaches (2 fruit)

Dinner
casserole of 3 oz baked cheddar and Swiss cheese (3 meat)
   with 1 cup of onions (2 vegetable)
Chinese cabbage (as desired)
1 cup boiled potatoes (2 bread)
1 sl whole wheat bread (1 bread)
1 tsp butter or margarine (1 fat)
1 cup watermelon (1 fruit)
1 cup skim milk (1 dairy)

Bedtime snack
2 dates (1 fruit)
9 rye wafers (3 bread)
½ cup skim milk (½ dairy)

THURSDAY

Breakfast
1 sl toast (1 bread)
1 piece angel or sponge cake (2 bread)
2 tsp butter or margarine (2 fat)
2 lge fresh figs (2 fruit)
1 cup skim milk (1 dairy)

Lunch
mushroom and pea omelet made with 2 eggs (2 meat), ½ cup
    skim milk (½ dairy), ½ cup peas (1 bread), and ½ cup
    mushrooms (1 vegetable)
2 sl whole wheat bread (1 bread)
1 tsp butter or margarine (1 fat)
1 muffin (1 bread)
1 lge peach (2 fruit)
1 cup skim milk (1 dairy)

Dinner
3 oz lean hamburger (3 meat)
1 roll (1 bread)
1 cup spaghetti with sauce (2 bread)
½ cup carrots (1 vegetable)
½ cup green and red peppers (1 vegetable)
lettuce (as desired)
1 tbsp dressing (1 fat)
1 peach (1 fruit)
1 cup skim milk (1 dairy)

Bedtime snack
6 graham crackers (3 bread)
½ cup grapefruit juice (1 fruit)

FRIDAY

Breakfast
¼ cup wheat germ (1 bread)
2 sl whole wheat toast (2 bread)
2 tsp butter or margarine (2 fat)
½ cantaloupe (2 fruit)
1 cup skim milk (1 dairy)

Lunch
2 oz lean pork chop (2 meat)
1 cup rice (2 bread)
½ cup peas (1 bread)
½ cup cooked beets (1 vegetable)
⅓ cup applesauce (1 fruit)
Chinese cabbage (as desired)
2 tsp lo-cal mayonnaise dressing (1 fat)
10 lge cherries (1 fruit)
1 cup skim milk (1 dairy)

Dinner
2 oz liver (2 meat)
1 cup mashed potatoes (2 bread)
1 oz shredded cheddar cheese to mix with potatoes (1 meat)
½ cup green beans (1 vegetable)
½ cup turnips (1 vegetable)
endive (as desired)
1 tbsp lo-cal Italian dressing (1 fat)
1 med orange (1 fruit)
1 cup skim milk (1 dairy)

Bedtime snack
1 lge piece angel or sponge cake (3 bread)
¾ cup mandarin oranges (1 fruit)

SATURDAY

Breakfast
1 cup flavored yogurt (1 dairy)
1 toasted bagel (2 bread)
2 tbsp cream cheese (2 fat)
⅛ honeydew melon (1 fruit)
½ cup grapefruit juice (1 fruit)

Lunch
3 fish sticks (1 bread, 2 meat)
2 sl whole wheat bread (2 bread)
1 tsp butter or margarine (1 fat)
½ cup winter squash (1 vegetable)
4 dates (2 fruit)
1 cup skim milk (1 dairy)

Dinner
10 med shrimp (3 meat)
lettuce (as desired)
2 tsp lo-cal mayonnaise (1 fat)
pinch of curry powder to add to mayo and pour over shrimp
½ cup sliced mushrooms (1 vegetable)
½ cup raw broccoli (1 vegetable)
2 tortillas (2 bread)
½ cup rice (1 bread)
2 lge plums (2 fruit)
1 cup skim milk (1 dairy)

Bedtime snack
12 saltines (2 bread)
¾ cup popcorn (1 bread)
¼ cup grape juice (1 fruit)

SUNDAY

Breakfast
½ cup vegetable juice cocktail, dash of Tabasco, Worcestershire
    sauce, stick of celery (1 vegetable)
1 sm grapefruit (2 fruit)
1½ English muffins (3 bread)
2 tsp butter or margarine (2 fat)
1 cup skim milk (1 dairy)

Lunch
crab sandwich
½ cup crab (2 meat)
2 tsp lo-cal mayonnaise (1 fat)
3 sl whole wheat bread (3 bread)
1 cup cucumber slices (1 vegetable)
¼ honeydew melon (2 fruit)

Dinner
3 oz lean roast lamb (3 meat)
mint sauce (to taste)
2 roast potatoes (2 bread)
½ cup peas (1 bread)
½ cup roast carrots (1 vegetable)
½ cup steamed cauliflower (1 vegetable)
1 dinner roll (1 bread)
1 tsp butter or margarine (1 fat)
1 sm nectarine (1 fruit)
1 cup skim milk (1 dairy)

Bedtime snack
¼ cantaloupe (1 fruit)
10 sm variety crackers (2 bread)

MONDAY

Breakfast
1 cup grapefruit juice (2 fruit)
1½ cups dry cereal (2 bread)
1 sl toast (1 bread)
1 tsp margarine or butter (1 fat)
1 cup skim milk (1 dairy) (can be used partly with cereal)

Lunch
ham and cheese sandwich
1 oz boiled ham (1 meat)
1 oz Swiss cheese (1 meat)
1 bun (2 bread)
1 tsp mayonnaise (1 fat)
1 muffin (1 bread)
1 med orange (2 fruit)
1 cup skim milk (1 dairy)

Dinner
fish 'n' chips
3 oz halibut (3 meat)
oil for frying (1 fat)
batter:
    2½ tbsp flour (1 bread)
    salt (or salt substitute) to taste
    pepper to taste
    ⅛ cup beer (plus water as desired)
2 potatoes, french-fried (2 bread, 1 fat)
½ cup sautéd mushrooms (1 vegetable)
½ cup boiled brussels sprouts (1 vegetable)
½ cup fruit cocktail (1 fruit)
1 cup skim milk (1 dairy)

Bedtime snack
3 matzoh wafers (3 bread)
⅓ cup apple juice (1 fruit)

TUESDAY

Breakfast
½ cup prune juice (2 fruit)
1 toasted bun (2 bread)
1 blueberry muffin (1 bread)
2 tsp butter or margarine (2 fat)
1 cup skim milk (1 dairy)

Lunch
tuna sandwich
½ cup water-packed tuna (2 meat)
3 sl whole wheat bread (3 bread)
2 tsp lo-cal mayonnaise (1 fat)
pepper to taste
½ cup celery sticks (1 vegetable)
lettuce (as desired)
4 med apricots (2 fruit)
1 cup skim milk (1 dairy)

Dinner
chicken omelet made with 1 oz grated chicken (1 meat), 2 eggs
    (2 meat), ½ cup peas (1 bread), ½ cup skim milk (½ dairy), and
    ½ cup diced mixed peppers (1 vegetable)
1 tsp margarine or butter to cook (1 fat)
3 boiled potatoes (3 bread)
½ cup asparagus (1 vegetable)
½ sm banana (1 fruit)
½ cup skim milk (½ dairy)

Bedtime snack
20 lge potato or corn chips (2 bread)
½ cup orange juice (1 fruit)

WEDNESDAY

Breakfast
1 cup grapefruit juice (2 fruit)
1 English muffin (2 bread)
1 egg (1 meat)
1 cup skim milk (1 dairy)

Lunch
egg sandwich
2 hard-boiled eggs (2 meat)
1 cubed boiled potato (1 bread)
2 tsp lo-cal mayonnaise (1 fat)
½ cup chopped celery (1 vegetable)
salt and pepper to taste
2 sl white bread (2 bread)
1 med apple (2 fruit)
1 cup skim milk (1 dairy)

Dinner
2 oz veal, sautéd (2 meat)
2 baked potatoes (2 bread)
2 tbsp sour cream (1 fat)
½ cup bean sprouts (1 vegetable)
½ cup green or yellow beans (1 vegetable)
1 med pear (2 fruit)
1 cup skim milk (1 dairy)

Bedtime snack
6 graham crackers (3 bread)
⅓ cup apple cider (1 fruit)

THURSDAY

Breakfast
1 cup plain yogurt (1 dairy)
1 cup blueberries (2 fruit)
1 toasted bagel (2 bread)
2 tsp butter (2 fat)
1 muffin (1 bread)

Lunch
open-faced grilled-cheese sandwich
2 sl whole grain bread (2 bread)
2 oz cheddar or Swiss cheese (2 meat)
½ cup sliced mushrooms (1 vegetable)
pepper to taste
¼ honeydew melon (2 fruit)
1 cup skim milk (1 dairy)

Dinner
beef kabob
3 oz cubed beef (3 meat)
¼ cup zucchini (½ vegetable)
¼ cup onions (½ vegetable)
¼ cup tomatoes (½ vegetable)
¼ cup summer squash (½ vegetable)
3 boiled potatoes (3 bread)
1 dinner roll (1 bread)
1 tsp butter or margarine (1 fat)
½ cup pineapple (1 fruit)
1 cup skim milk (1 dairy)

Bedtime snack
½ cup ice cream (1 bread, 2 fat)
6 rye wafers (2 bread)
12 grapes (1 fruit)

FRIDAY

Breakfast
1 muffin (1 bread)
1 cup orange juice (2 fruit)
1½ cups dry cereal (2 bread)
1 cup skim milk (1 dairy)

Lunch
shrimp sandwich
10 sm shrimp (2 meat)
3 sl whole wheat bread (3 bread)
2 tsp lo-cal mayonnaise (1 fat)
½ cup sliced cucumbers (1 vegetable)
1 med nectarine (2 fruit)
1 cup skim milk (1 dairy)

Dinner
3 oz liver, sautéd (3 meat)
1 cup sautéd onions (2 vegetables)
½ cup brussels sprouts (1 vegetable)
1 cup savory rice (2 bread)
1 dinner roll (1 bread)
1 tsp butter or margarine (1 fat)
¾ cup strawberries (1 fruit)
1 cup skim milk (1 dairy)

Bedtime snack
1 toasted English muffin (2 bread)
2 graham crackers (1 bread)
⅓ cup pineapple juice (1 fruit)

SATURDAY

Breakfast
3 sl whole wheat toast (3 bread)
2 tsp butter or margarine (2 fat)
1 med grapefruit (2 fruit)
1 cup skim milk (1 dairy)

Lunch
1 poached egg (1 meat)
1 oz boiled ham (1 meat)
1 English muffin (2 bread)
2 tbsp lo-cal mayonnaise (1 fat)
½ cup asparagus (1 vegetable)
1 sm piece angel cake (1 bread)
1 cup fruit salad (2 fruit)
1 cup skim milk (1 dairy)

Dinner
3 oz roast pork (3 meat)
2 roast potatoes (2 bread)
1 dinner roll (1 bread)
½ cup steamed cauliflower (1 vegetable)
½ cup beets (1 vegetable)
½ cup applesauce (1 fruit)
1 cup skim milk (1 dairy)

Bedtime snack
20 lge potato chips (2 bread)
6 pretzels (1 bread)
½ cup orange juice (1 fruit)

SUNDAY

Breakfast
½ cup vegetable juice cocktail (1 vegetable)
1 med grapefruit (2 fruit)
2 pieces corn bread (2 bread)
2 tsp butter or margarine (2 fat)
1 cup skim milk (1 dairy)

Lunch
3 med sardines (1 meat)
1 oz chunk strong cheese (1 meat)
French toast
1 egg (1 meat)
3 sl whole wheat bread (3 bread)
4 dates (2 fruit)
1 cup skim milk (1 dairy)

Dinner
2 sm oysters, sautéd (⅓ meat)
2 sm clams, sautéd (⅓ meat)
2 sm scallops, sautéd (⅓ meat)
5 sm shrimp, sautéd (1 meat)
pepper, salt, paprika, dash of lemon juice to taste
1 tbsp thick cream (1 fat)
pinches of flour to thicken if necessary
¼ cup sweet potatoes (1 bread)
2 boiled potatoes (2 bread)
½ cup asparagus (1 vegetable)
½ cup carrots (1 vegetable)
½ cup broccoli (1 vegetable)
1 sm banana (2 fruit)
1 cup skim milk (1 dairy)

Bedtime snack
3 sl raisin bread (3 bread)
⅓ cup pineapple juice (1 fruit)

3,000 CALORIES (approx)

A simple way to follow the 3,000 calorie regimen is to base it on this table:

Breakfast
3 fruit exchanges
4 bread exchanges
2 fat exchanges
1 dairy exchange

Midmorning snack
2 bread exchanges
½ dairy exchange

Lunch
3 meat exchanges
4 bread exchanges
3 fat exchanges
2 vegetable exchanges
2 fruit exchanges
1 dairy exchange

Midafternoon snack
2 bread exchanges
1 fruit exchange

Dinner
4 meat exchanges
4 bread exchanges
2 vegetable exchanges
vegetables (unrestricted) as desired
1 fruit exchange
2 fat exchanges
1 dairy exchange

Bedtime snack
3 bread exchanges
1 fat exchange
1 fruit exchange

―――――――――――――― **MONDAY** ――――――――――――

Breakfast
1 cup orange juice (2 fruit)
2 tbsp raisins (1 fruit)
1 English muffin (2 bread)
2 tsp butter or margarine (2 fat)
1 cup cooked cereal (2 bread)
1 cup skim milk (1 dairy)

Midmorning snack
12 saltines (2 bread)
½ cup skim milk (½ dairy)

Lunch
3½ oz cold cuts (3 meat)
4 sl whole wheat bread (4 bread)
3 tsp mayonnaise (3 fat)
½ cup celery sticks (1 vegetable)
½ cup raw carrots (1 vegetable)
radishes (as desired)
1 med orange (2 fruit)
1 cup skim milk (1 dairy)

Midafternoon snack
2 corn muffins (2 bread)
10 cherries (1 fruit)

Dinner
4 oz baked ham (4 meat)
1 cup peas (2 bread)

2 boiled potatoes (2 bread)
1 dinner roll (1 bread)
1 cup tomatoes (2 vegetable)
lettuce (as desired)
½ cup fruit cocktail (1 fruit)
2 tsp butter or margarine (2 fat)
1 cup skim milk (1 dairy)

Bedtime snack
2 sl raisin bread (2 bread)
1 tsp butter (1 fat)
3 rye wafers (1 bread)
⅓ cup apple juice (1 fruit)

TUESDAY

Breakfast
2 sl French bread (2 bread)
2 corn muffins (2 bread)
2 tsp butter (2 fat)
1 cup grapefruit juice (2 fruit)
½ sm banana (1 fruit)
1 cup skim milk (1 dairy)

Midmorning snack
4 graham crackers (2 bread)
½ cup skim milk (½ dairy)

Lunch
cheese and onion omelet
2 eggs (2 meat)
1 oz cheddar cheese (1 meat)
½ cup diced onions (1 vegetable)
½ cup bean sprouts (1 vegetable)
salt, pepper, paprika to season
2 sl whole wheat bread (2 bread)
2 tsp butter for bread (2 fat)

1 tsp butter for omelet (1 fat)
1 cup savory rice (2 bread)
2 plums (2 fruit)
1 cup skim milk (1 dairy)

Midafternoon snack
2 raisin muffins (2 bread)
½ cup orange juice (1 fruit)

Dinner
½ cup cottage cheese (2 meat)
½ cup crab (2 meat)
2 tortillas (2 bread)
2 tsp mayonnaise (2 fat)
½ cup cold green beans (1 vegetable)
½ cup uncooked cauliflower (1 vegetable)
½ cup cold peas (1 bread)
1 dinner roll (1 bread)
1 sm piece sponge cake (1 bread)
1 lge tangerine (1 fruit)
1 cup skim milk (1 dairy)

Bedtime snack
½ cup sherbet (2 bread)
1 sl whole grain toast (1 bread)
1 tsp butter (1 fat)
¼ cup grape juice (1 fruit)

WEDNESDAY

Breakfast
1 cup yogurt (1 dairy)
1 cup blueberries (2 fruit)
1 toasted English muffin (2 bread)
1 bagel (2 bread)
2 tsp butter (2 fat)
½ cup grapefruit juice (1 fruit)

Midmorning snack
1 cup dry cereal (2 bread)
½ cup skim milk (½ dairy)

Lunch
tuna and celery sandwich
¾ cup tuna (3 meat)
3 tsp mayonnaise (3 fat)
4 sl whole wheat bread (4 bread)
1 cup chopped celery (2 vegetable)
1 lge peach (2 fruit)
1 cup skim milk (1 dairy)

Midafternoon snack
2 corn muffins (2 bread)
1 sm apple (1 fruit)

Dinner
breaded and fried chicken (no skin) made with 3 oz chicken
    pieces (3 meat), 3 tbsp breadcrumbs (1 bread), 1 egg
    (1 meat), and salt and pepper to taste
1 tsp butter for frying chicken (1 fat)
1 cup grits (2 bread)
2 sl bread (2 bread)
1 tsp butter (1 fat)
Lettuce (as desired)
½ cup spinach (1 vegetable)
½ cup turnips (1 vegetable)
12 grapes (1 fruit)
1 cup skim milk (1 dairy)

Bedtime snack
1 lge piece angel cake (3 bread)
¾ cup papaya (1 fruit)

THURSDAY

Breakfast
¼ avocado (2 fat)
1 cup orange juice (2 fruit)
2 dates (1 fruit)
3 muffins (3 bread)
½ cup skim milk (½ dairy)

Midmorning snack
1 toasted English muffin (2 bread)
2 graham crackers (1 bread)
1 cup skim milk (1 dairy)

Lunch
shrimp salad
15 sm shrimp (3 meat)
3 sl whole wheat bread
3 tsp butter (3 fat)
lettuce (as desired)
½ cup chopped raw carrots (1 vegetable)
½ cup bean sprouts (1 vegetable)
1 med apple (2 fruit)
1 cup skim milk (1 dairy)

Midafternoon snack
1 med piece sponge cake (2 bread)
1 sm pear (1 fruit)

Dinner
beef kabob
4 oz chunked beef (4 meat)
¼ cup zucchini (½ vegetable)
¼ cup tomatoes (½ vegetable)
¼ cup onions (½ vegetable)
¼ cup asparagus (½ vegetable)
2 sl whole wheat bread (2 bread)
1 cup peas (2 bread)

1 baked potato (1 bread)
2 tsp butter (2 fat)
¼ cantaloupe (1 fruit)
1 cup skim milk (1 dairy)

Bedtime snack
2 sl toasted French bread (2 bread)
1 sl raisin bread (1 bread)
1 tsp butter (1 fat)
1 sm orange (1 fruit)

FRIDAY

Breakfast
1 cup plain yogurt (1 dairy)
1 cup raspberries (2 fruit)
⅓ cup apple juice (1 fruit)
3 sl whole grain toast (3 bread)
1 corn muffin (1 bread)
2 tsp butter (2 fat)

Midmorning snack
1½ cups popcorn (1 bread)
6 pretzels (1 bread)
½ cup skim milk (½ dairy)

Lunch
open-faced grilled-cheese sandwich
2 sl whole grain bread (2 bread)
3 oz cheddar cheese (3 meat)
½ cup mushrooms (1 vegetable)
½ cup tomatoes (1 vegetable)
2 tbsp cream cheese (2 fat)
4 fresh apricots (2 fruit)
1 cup skim milk (1 dairy)

Midafternoon snack
2 blueberry muffins (2 bread)
½ cup grapefruit juice (1 fruit)

Dinner
4 oz lean lamb chops (4 meat)
3 boiled potatoes (3 bread)
parsley for garnish
mint sauce (not jelly)
½ cup brussels sprouts (1 vegetable)
½ cup summer squash (1 vegetable)
2 sl whole wheat bread (2 bread)
2 tsp butter (2 fat)
1 med peach (1 fruit)
1 cup skim milk (1 dairy)

Bedtime snack
4 graham crackers (2 bread)
1 sl whole wheat toast (1 bread)
1 tsp butter (1 fat)
½ cup orange juice (1 fruit)

SATURDAY

Breakfast
1 cup grapefruit juice (2 fruit)
2 tbsp raisins (1 fruit)
1½ cups dry cereal (2 bread)
1 toasted bagel (2 bread)
2 tsp butter (2 fat)
1 cup skim milk (1 dairy)

Midmorning snack
2 corn muffins (2 bread)
½ cup skim milk (½ dairy)

Lunch
salmon salad
¾ cup salmon (3 meat)
lettuce (as desired)
2 sl French bread (2 bread)
1 tsp butter (1 fat)
2 tbsp French dressing (2 fat)
½ cup chopped celery (1 vegetable)
½ cup raw cabbage (1 vegetable)
1 sm banana (2 fruit)
1 cup skim milk (1 dairy)

Midafternoon snack
½ cup wheat germ (2 bread)
½ sm mango (1 fruit)

Dinner
4 oz roast beef (4 meat)
3 roast potatoes (3 bread)
2 dinner rolls (2 bread)
2 tsp butter (2 fat)
lettuce and radishes (as desired)
½ cup turnips (1 vegetable)
½ cup steamed broccoli (1 vegetable)
10 lge cherries (1 fruit)
1 cup skim milk (1 dairy)

Bedtime snack
1 cup rice (2 bread)
3 rye wafers (1 bread)
½ cup grapefruit juice (1 fruit)

—————————————— **SUNDAY** ——————————————

Breakfast
1 cup buttermilk (1 dairy)
1 toasted English muffin (2 bread)

2 blueberry muffins (2 bread)
2 tsp butter (2 fat)
½ cup prune juice (2 fruit)
1 sm orange (1 fruit)

Midmorning snack
1 med piece sponge cake (2 bread)
½ cup skim milk (½ dairy)

Lunch
3 oz cold cuts (3 meat)
4 sl whole wheat bread (4 bread)
3 tsp mayonnaise (3 fat)
1 cup celery sticks (2 vegetable)
1 med nectarine (2 fruit)
1 cup skim milk (1 dairy)

Midafternoon snack
2 sl raisin bread (2 bread)
⅓ cup apple juice (1 fruit)

Dinner
4 oz roast turkey (4 meat)
½ cup savory stuffing (2 bread)
½ cup peas (1 bread)
1 baked potato (1 bread)
1 dinner roll (1 bread)
1 tsp butter (1 fat)
½ cup turnips (1 vegetable)
½ cup green beans (1 vegetable)
1 cup watermelon (1 fruit)
1 cup skim milk (1 dairy)

Bedtime snack
½ cup strawberry ice cream (1 bread, 2 fat)
1 med piece angel cake (2 bread)
½ cup orange juice (1 fruit)

——— MONDAY ———

Breakfast
1 grapefruit (2 fruit)
1 cup hot cereal (2 bread)
2 sl whole grain toast (2 bread)
2 tsp butter (2 fat)
1 cup skim milk (1 dairy)

Midmorning snack
2 corn muffins (2 bread)
½ cup skim milk (½ dairy)

Lunch
baked sole
3 oz sole in casserole (3 meat)
1 cup buttermilk (1 dairy)
pepper to taste
2 boiled potatoes (2 bread)
2 sl whole wheat bread (2 bread)
2 tsp butter (2 fat)
lettuce (as desired)
½ cup baked eggplant (1 vegetable)
½ cup boiled beets (1 vegetable)
¼ honeydew melon (2 fruits)

Midafternoon snack
20 lge potato chips (2 bread)
⅓ cup apple cider (1 fruit)

Dinner
ham, cheese, and onion omelet
1 oz chopped ham (1 meat)
1 oz grated cheddar cheese (1 meat)
2 eggs (2 meat)
½ cup buttermilk (½ dairy)
salt, pepper, paprika, onion powder to taste
2 dinner rolls (2 bread)

2 tsp butter (2 fat)
1 cup mashed potatoes (2 bread)
½ cup peas (1 bread)
½ cup steamed cauliflower (1 vegetable)
½ cup turnips (1 vegetable)
1 sm orange (1 fruit)
½ cup skim milk (½ dairy)

Bedtime snack
2 blueberry muffins (2 bread)
1 sl toast (1 bread)
1 tsp butter (1 fat)
¼ cup grape juice (1 fruit)

TUESDAY

Breakfast
1 med grapefruit (2 fruit)
⅓ cup apple juice (1 fruit)
1 toasted English muffin (2 bread)
2 tsp butter (2 fat)
1 corn muffin (1 bread)
1 cup skim milk (1 dairy)

Midmorning snack
1 lge piece sponge cake (3 bread)
½ cup skim milk (½ dairy)

Lunch
crab sandwich
3 oz crab meat (3 meat)
4 tbsp lo-cal mayonnaise (2 fat)
4 sl whole wheat bread (4 bread)
1 cup cucumber slices (2 vegetable)
¼ honeydew melon (2 fruit)
1 cup skim milk (1 dairy)

Midafternoon snack
Jell-O mold
¼ cup fruit-flavored gelatin
½ cup fruit salad (1 fruit)

Dinner
chef's salad
2 oz shredded Swiss cheese (2 meat)
2 oz chopped boiled ham (2 meat)
lettuce and ½ cup raw veg (1 vegetable)
1 med tomato sliced (1 vegetable)
2 tbsp dressing (2 fat)
1 cup spaghetti with sauce (3 bread)
2 dinner rolls (2 bread)
½ cup orange juice (1 fruit)
1 cup skim milk (1 dairy)

Bedtime snack
2 sl toasted raisin bread (2 bread)
1 corn muffin (1 bread)
1 tsp butter (1 fat)
½ cup grapefruit juice (1 fruit)

─────────────── **WEDNESDAY** ───────────────

Breakfast
1½ cups fruit cocktail (3 fruit)
1 toasted bagel (2 bread)
2 tsp butter (2 fat)
1 muffin (1 bread)
1 cup skim milk (1 dairy)

Midmorning snack
1 lge ear corn on the cob (3 bread)
½ cup skim milk (½ dairy)

Lunch
3 fish sticks (1 bread, 2 meat)
⅔ cup parsnips (1 bread)
2 sl whole wheat bread (2 bread)
3 tsp butter (3 fat)
1 cup sautéd mushrooms (2 vegetable)
1 cup watermelon (1 fruit)
⅓ cup apple juice (1 fruit)
1 cup skim milk (1 dairy)

Midafternoon snack
1 muffin (1 bread)
10 lge corn chips (1 bread)
½ cup orange juice (1 fruit)

Dinner
4 oz lean steak (4 meat)
1 cup mashed potatoes (2 bread)
2 dinner rolls (2 bread)
2 tsp butter (2 fat)
½ cup cabbage (1 vegetable)
½ cup green beans (1 vegetable)
1 7-oz glass ginger ale (1 bread)
lettuce (as desired)
½ cup pineapple (1 fruit)
1 cup skim milk (1 dairy)

Bedtime snack
2 muffins (2 bread)
1 sl toast (1 bread)
1 tsp butter (1 fat)
½ cup pineapple juice (1 fruit)

THURSDAY

Breakfast
1 sl crisp bacon (1 fat)
2 sl raisin bread (2 bread)
2 tsp butter (2 fat)
1 cup hot cereal (2 bread)
½ cup orange juice (1 fruit)
2 dates (1 fruit)
1 cup skim milk (1 dairy)

Midmorning snack
2 muffins (2 bread)
½ cup skim milk (½ dairy)

Lunch
6 Vienna sausages (3 meat)
2 buns (4 bread)
2 tsp butter or mayonnaise (2 fat)
½ cup asparagus (1 vegetable)
½ cup bean sprouts (1 vegetable)
1 med pear (2 fruit)
1 cup skim milk (1 dairy)

Midafternoon snack
20 lge potato chips (2 bread)
½ sm grapefruit (1 fruit)

Dinner
15 med shrimp (4 meat)
lettuce (as desired)
½ cup raw mushrooms (1 vegetable)
½ cup raw carrots (1 vegetable)
4 tbsp lo-cal mayonnaise (2 fat)
3 tortillas (3 bread)
1 cup rice (2 bread)
2 med plums (1 fruit)
1 cup skim milk (1 dairy)

Bedtime snack
½ cup wheat germ (2 bread)
1 sl whole wheat toast (1 bread)
1 tsp butter (1 fat)
⅓ cup apple cider (1 fruit)

─────────────── **FRIDAY** ───────────────

Breakfast
1 boiled egg (1 meat)
3 sl whole wheat toast (3 bread)
2 tsp butter (2 fat)
1 corn muffin (1 bread)
1 med grapefruit (2 fruit)
2 tbsp raisins (1 fruit)
1 cup skim milk (1 dairy)

Midmorning snack
1 med piece angel cake (2 bread)
½ cup skim milk (½ dairy)

Lunch
omelet
1 egg (1 meat)
1 oz grated cheddar cheese (1 meat)
1 cup grits (2 bread)
2 sl whole wheat bread (2 bread)
2 tsp butter (2 fat)
1 cup brussels sprouts (2 vegetable)
½ cup fruit cocktail (1 fruit)
10 lge cherries (1 fruit)
1 cup skim milk (1 dairy)

Midafternoon snack
1 toasted English muffin (2 bread)
1 tsp butter (1 fat)
½ cup orange juice (1 fruit)

Dinner
4 oz lean hamburger for meatballs (4 meat)
1½ cups spaghetti and sauce (3 bread)
½ cup carrots (1 vegetable)
½ cup broccoli (1 vegetable)
1 dinner roll (1 bread)
1 tsp butter (1 fat)
¾ cup strawberries (1 fruit)
1 cup skim milk (1 dairy)

Bedtime snack
4 graham crackers (2 bread)
1 English muffin (2 bread)
1 tsp butter (1 fat)
¼ cup prune juice (1 fruit)

———————— SATURDAY ————————

Breakfast
½ cantaloupe (2 fruit)
½ cup orange juice (1 fruit)
1 toasted bagel (2 bread)
2 tsp butter (2 fat)
1 muffin (1 bread)
1 cup skim milk (1 dairy)

Midmorning snack
½ cup celery sticks (1 vegetable)
1 med piece sponge cake (2 bread)
½ cup skim milk (½ dairy)

Lunch
¾ cup salmon (3 meat)
4 sl whole wheat bread (4 bread)
3 tsp mayonnaise (3 fat)
½ cup sliced cucumbers (1 vegetable)

24 grapes (2 fruit)
1 cup skim milk (1 dairy)

Midafternoon snack
12 pretzels (2 bread)
1 sm orange (1 fruit)

Dinner
20 sm clams (4 meat)
1 tbsp light cream for sautéing clams (1 fat)
pepper to taste
2 tbsp flour to mix with clams and cream (1 bread)
⅔ cup parsnips (1 bread)
½ cup peas (1 bread)
2 dinner rolls (2 bread)
2 tsp butter (2 fat)
lettuce and radishes (as desired)
1 cup steamed cauliflower (2 vegetable)
1 sm apple (1 fruit)
1 cup skim milk (1 dairy)

Bedtime snack
6 rye wafers (2 bread)
1 sl whole wheat toast (1 bread)
1 tsp butter (1 fat)
¼ cup grape juice (1 fruit)

————————————— **SUNDAY** —————————————

Breakfast
½ cup chocolate ice cream (1 bread, 2 fat)
1 cup hot cereal (2 bread)
1 sm piece angel cake (1 bread)
1 med peach (1 fruit)
2 tbsp raisins (1 fruit)
1 cup skim milk (1 dairy)

Midmorning snack
1½ cups popcorn (1 bread)
6 saltines (1 bread)
½ cup skim milk (½ dairy)

Lunch
6 med sardines (2 meat)
1 hard-boiled egg (1 meat)
1 cup savory rice (2 bread)
2 tortillas (2 bread)
2 tbsp sour cream (2 fat)
⅛ avocado (1 fat)
½ cup green and red peppers (1 vegetable)
½ cup sliced cucumbers (1 vegetable)
1 cup watermelon (1 fruit)
½ cup boysenberries (1 fruit)
1 cup skim milk (1 dairy)

Midafternoon snack
10 sm variety crackers (2 bread)
½ sm banana (1 fruit)

Dinner
4 oz roast beef (4 meat)
3 roast potatoes (3 bread)
½ cup peas (1 bread)
½ cup turnips (1 vegetable) plus 1 tsp butter (1 fat)
½ cup green beans (1 vegetable)
1 dinner roll (1 bread)
1 tsp butter (1 fat)
¾ cup papaya (1 fruit)
1 cup skim milk (1 dairy)

Bedtime snack
¼ cup fruit-flavored gelatin
½ cup fruit cocktail (1 fruit)
1 sl whole wheat toast (1 bread)

1 tsp butter (1 fat)
1 sm piece angel cake (1 bread)

TEMPTING TASTE TIPS

Certain herbs and spices can add a whole new taste dimension to a meal. There are numerous ways you can add zest to the meals you cook, and also some handy tips for cooking and preparing.

Flavor Enhancers

MEATS: bay leaves, sage, dry mustard, parsley, oregano, onion, green pepper, lemon juice, paprika, thyme, marjoram, curry powder, rosemary, turmeric.

EGGS: curry powder, dry mustard, tomato, parsley, green pepper, mushrooms, onions, turmeric.

VEGETABLES: chives, dill, fennel, pimento strips, garlic, onion juice, lemon juice, teriyaki sauce, soy sauce, dill, mace, parsley, marjoram, basil, plain yogurt, buttermilk.

RICE: powdered soup mixes are excellent to add to rice; while it's cooking, turn it into a savory special.

SALADS: unflavored gelatin together with vegetable juices and raw vegetables make wonderful salads.

DRESSINGS: low-calorie dressings can be produced by using vinegar, pickle juice, tomato juice, yogurt, or lemon juice as a base. For even more different flavors you can add seasoned salt, pepper, garlic, dill, tarragon, paprika, and dry mustard.

10

AN EASY START
TO THE DIET

In our studies involving pain among outpatients at Temple University, one point has become all too obvious: Many pain victims are seriously malnourished. This is not to say that they are walking skeletons; in some cases they are quite the opposite. What it does mean is that these people have let their nutritional values slip; they have been eating many of the wrong foods and in undesirable combinations.

The sad fact with chronic and acute pain is that they have a severe demoralizing effect on the victim. We have already seen the connection between pain and depression, and unfortunately this syndrome can have far-reaching effects, especially in the diet.

When a person is in pain and depressed, one of the first things that begins to slide is nutrition. If you're relying heavily on painkilling drugs, this again can dull your appetite and lead to bad eating habits.

Fast foods and junk foods often seem the easiest and simplest way to serve your daily nutritional needs. With the pain victim these types of foods often appear more attractive because they are easily accessible and take little or no time to prepare. (We are talking about the fast-food hamburgers and fries, pizzas, hot sandwiches, quick Mexican tacos, and the like.) It's often just a question of throwing them into a microwave or the oven to reheat.

Depression is another key factor on this nutritional downhill slide. In our clinical experience with pain victims, depression can drain any hope of well-being; patients don't give up totally on life, but they begin to let the quality of life slip: There's a feeling of "What's the point?", "Why should I care?" To them, eating is simply a method of satisfying occasional hunger pangs, and just about whatever food that comes within arm's reach will serve the purpose.

The opposite are the binge eaters. These people will gorge themselves on anything and everything as they seek a false pacifier in food for their pain and depression. Unfortunately, their gargantuan meals are often made up of junk and snack foods that hold very little nutritional value. Naturally, these people tend to be overweight, and despite their obvious bulk they can still be nutritionally undernourished. And we know that excess weight can inflame an already painful condition.

It's truly a vicious cycle: When pain and depression detract from sensible eating habits and good nutrition, the body's resources for combating pain become depleted. Thus the pain and depression worsen, and food intake may become even more erratic on this downhill spiral.

There is no instant solution to this problem because bad eating habits tend to die hard. Once the body has fallen out of good nutritional balance it may take some time for it to come around to accepting and enjoying a nutritionally optimum diet.

For many pain sufferers, returning to a sound nutritional balance is a major task in itself. But one approach we have found to be successful is to gradually wean the undernourished back into the mainstream of sensible eating by utilizing high-nutrition formulas as substitutes for some meals at the start of the Pain-Free Diet.

You might wish to use this technique as an easy and

invigorating alternate way to starting the Pain-Free Diet plan. The object is to bring your body quickly and safely back into nutritional balance by alternating your own prepared meals from the diet with meals of snacks made from the high-nutrition formulas.

NUTRITION-BOOSTING FORMULAS

These high-nutrition formulas are mostly powdered mixes that are blended with milk or water to produce tasty (and sometimes not so tasty) meal substitutes which are drunk instead of eaten. What most of these commercial formulas have in common is that they are aimed at quick weight loss on diet programs while providing the body with the nutrients (protein, carbohydrate, fat, vitamins, and minerals) essential for health. What they also have in common is that they supply these needs at extremely low caloric levels— the object being to burn off excess calories already present in fat tissue. Because the body needs more calories than these products supply each day, it reaches into its reserves of fat and uses these calories for energy.

This all looks very sound, but these types of diet formulas have a tendency to be abused. The only safe weight loss is one that is gradual. Many of these formulas are accompanied by instructions that promote rapid weight loss: too much, too soon! This can be dangerous when followed for any extended period of time. These formulas are designed to appeal to the overweight because of their simplicity and ease, and promise of quick results.

One of the most commercially prominent of these diets is the Cambridge Plan™, and if imitation is a sure sign of success, Cambridge must be doing something right for many thousands of overweight people. Since its introduction in the United States, the Cambridge Plan has been the single source of inspiration for many imitators who obviously also want a bite of the overweight pie and its potentially huge profits.

Cambridge and many other diet formulas do provide a unique and sensible balance of essential nutrients, but at the expense of an unnervingly low daily caloric intake. For example, the suggested daily three meals of early Cambridge formulas supplied a total of 330 calories, 33 grams of protein, 44 grams of carbohydrate, and 3 grams of fat. Three hundred and thirty calories a day is a dangerously low intake. Cambridge, however, has since modified its formulas to provide up to 800 calories a day from four servings and 100 percent of the RDAs, including calcium.

But Cambridge does stress the importance on all its formula container labels of consulting your physician before undertaking the diet plan. It also warns, "The Cambridge Diet formula is designed for use as a sole source of nutrition for periods not to exceed four consecutive weeks at any one time."

Although the caloric levels of Cambridge, and similar powdered and flavored diet products, are low, they do contain a highly desirable balance of protein, carbohydrate, and fat, plus the addition of essential vitamins and minerals. It is because of these beneficial aspects that we have found them to be successful adjuncts to starting the Pain-Free Diet—especially for people who have fallen into bad eating habits and are in need of a quick, safe, and effective nutritional boost.

HOW TO UTILIZE THE FORMULA APPROACH

The first thing you must be aware of when beginning the Pain-Free Diet using formulas is that they are being utilized solely as a starter. In no way should this either constitute

100 percent of your daily nutritional intake or be used longer than is necessary for you to return to "normal" eating habits. We do strongly suggest that if you are taking the formula approach to starting the diet, you should also advise your physician of the fact.

There is nothing wrong with formula drinks as nutrition-boosting snacks, or even as a replacement for the odd, occasional, missed meal. Because you are already aware of the low caloric content of the majority of formula products, you will be able to use your own discretion as to when it is likely to benefit your personally formulated Pain-Free Diet plan once it is in progress.

Another point to remember is that although these products give you a full 100 percent of the RDAs for vitamins and minerals, the best way to interpret the meaning of the RDAs is to remember that they are the minimum levels suggested for maintaining good health.

What is there to choose among formula products? The simple answer is not much! We can suggest Cambridge and another product, Twinsport Endurance B-Slim (more about the exact nutritional contents of both products shortly), because of their unique balance of protein, carbohydrate, and fat that closely follows the recommended balanced protein, increased-carbohydrate, and low-fat levels of the Pain-Free Diet plan.

To begin the formula-based introduction to the Pain-Free Diet, utilize the formula as a substitute for two main meals for the first three days. Breakfast and lunch are ideal because they will help to set up your system for a complete meal at dinner time, one that has been selected from the Pain-Free menu plans.

The formula can also be used as a substitute for midmorning or midafternoon snacks without substantially altering the weight-loss aspects of the program. You will still be taking your tryptophan-vitamin combinations with each meal whether it is formula or regular fare from the diet.

On the fourth day of utilizing the formula, substitute only

one main meal (preferably breakfast) and continue with this plan for the next five days. You will notice that if you have been having a problem with lack of appetite, this will be returning and you will actually be looking forward to those tasty fuller meals once more. For those of you who have been fighting binges, the gradually returning healthier nutritional balance will counteract this urge.

After nine or ten days using the formula substitution your body should become accustomed, easily and without stress, to accepting and thoroughly enjoying good nutritious and wholesome meals. You will experience a new feeling of well-being and a more relaxed and vibrant you.

When you discontinue the formula as a replacement for full meals, you can, if you wish, use it to replace daily snacks or missed meals.

FORMULA FORMULAS

Formula meals come in a variety of different flavors, most notably vanilla, chocolate, and strawberry. It is a matter of personal preference which one you choose.

The advantage of powdered formulas is that they can be mixed with water for a lower caloric content, or with milk for increased calories. The choice is yours, and the powdered formulas allow much more room for control, experimentation, and variety over premixed formulas.

The following nutritional contents of the two well-known commercial formulas we previously mentioned are listed as examples of both water- and milk-based products. If you do use a formula calling for milk and you already know you have a lactose intolerance, use milk products that have already had the lactose content either removed or broken down into a more digestible form.

Twinsport™ Endurance B-Slim® Meal
Replacement and Weight Control Formula

Manufacturer:
Twinsport, Inc.
2120 Smithtown Ave.
Ronkonkoma, NY 11779
(516) 467–3140

Contents (% of RDAs per serving):

vitamin A	25%
vitamin C	30%
vitamin B_1 (thiamine)	35%
vitamin B_2 (riboflavin)	10%
vitamin B_3 (niacin)	35%
vitamin B_6	30%
vitamin B_{12}	20%
vitamin D	10%
vitamin E	35%
biotin	35%
pantothenic acid	25%
calcium	15%
iron	35%
folic acid	20%
phosphorus	15%
iodine	35%
magnesium	25%
zinc	30%
copper	35%
manganese	1 mg*
potassium	240 mg*
chromium	10 mcg*
selenium	10 mcg*
molybdenum	10 mcg*

Flavors: chocolate and vanilla
Each serving, to be mixed with 8 oz low-fat milk, supplies:

calories	190
protein	15 gm

carbohydrate .... 31 gm
fat.. 1 gm
dietary fiber .... 2 gm

Note: Available through health food stores.

No RDAs established.

Cambridge 800 Diet

Manufacturer:
Cambridge Plan International
Salinas, CA 93901

Contents (% of RDAs per serving):
vitamin A.. 25%
vitamin C.. 25%
vitamin D.. 25%
vitamin E 25%
vitamin B_6 .... 25%
vitamin B_{12}.. 25%
thiamine 25%
riboflavin... 25%
niacin 25%
calcium.. 25%
iron.. 25%
folic acid 25%
phosphorus 25%
iodine 25%
magnesium 25%
zinc.. 25%
copper... 25%
biotin 25%
pantothenic acid.. 25%
vitamin K.. 16.7 mcg*
sodium... 375 mg*
potassium... 502.5 mg*
manganese... 1 mg*

chloride.. 450 mg*
chromium... 15 mcg*
selenium .... 15 mcg*
molybdenum... 37.5 mcg*

Flavors: vanilla, chocolate, strawberry
Each serving, mixed with water, supplies:
calories 200
protein.. 13 gm
carbohydrate .... 29 gm
fat.. 4 gm

Note: Cambridge products are supplied only through coun-
selors and are not available in stores.

*No RDAs established.

TASTY FORMULA TIPS

Even though manufacturers make formula products in a
variety of flavors, one of the biggest drawbacks is still the
lack of food "feeling." This stems from an aesthetic point
of view, mainly because of the repetitive consistency of the
mixed product. But by following a few simple tips you can
add further zest to formula products.

More calories. These can easily be obtained by using the
ice cream method or utilizing higher fat-content milks.

Additional Flavors. Baking essences and extracts are a snap
for providing additional flavors. You can experiment with
ones like mint, chocolate, cinnamon, etc.
Another idea is to add items like instant coffee mixes and
cocoa, and baking flavorings such as ground cinnamon.

Thicker mix. This can be achieved simply by adding a glass of ice to the mix and blending in a blender.

Another way is to mix a scoop of ice cream into the mix in the blender (but this also adds calories and fats—refer to the exchange lists for exactly how much).

The formula can also be premixed and left to partially set in a freezer for a few minutes.

11
HINTS TO HELP YOU STAY ON YOUR DIET

You may have tried to diet before and found it a frustrating experience. Two of the main reasons people fall off their diet plans are because either they lack the motivation or the diet has an adverse effect on them.

With the Pain-Free Diet you will not suffer any physical problems if you follow the diet plan carefully and pay attention to the chapter on eliminating foods that may be causing your pain problems. Remember, some of these maladies may have been the very reason that you abandoned previous diet attempts.

Once you have spent a few days on the diet you should be experiencing reduced or eliminated pain, a certain feeling of relaxation, and an increased awareness of health and well-being. These results in themselves should be more than enough to spur you on to continue with this beneficial nutritional regimen, whether you need to lose weight or not.

Because the Pain-Free Diet is a nutritional approach that you will customize to your own specific needs, you can even modify its weight-loss aspects to accommodate the occasional binge or splurge, and it's a good idea to do this as a reward to yourself once in a while.

But maybe your problem has always been motivation, the willpower needed to take the first step toward starting a diet that provides better nutrition and health.

As we've already pointed out, most people are not grossly overweight, but it's those few extra pounds that quite often make the difference between looking and feeling really healthy. If your physical looks alone don't trigger you to start the diet, the pain-free results certainly should.

If you are embarking on any important lifestyle change, we feel that preparation is very important and can help ease the transition between your present pain, weight, and health problems and optimum health. This is why we have included some psychological and practical tips designed to help trigger the Pain-Free Diet experience, followed by additional hints that will help you stick to it. We've also included some pointers for your spouse or friends to follow to contribute to your efforts and ensure your success.

DIET-TRIGGERING TIPS

A Positive Mental Attitude

Don't think of what you'll be giving up with your new diet; constantly remind yourself of what you are going to gain from it. Never feel sorry for yourself or let others be condescending toward your diet, but think of it as a new, improved lifestyle.

Reinforce Your Willpower

Before you start the diet, remember that you have just as much willpower as the next person. The more you think about your own willpower, the stronger it will become.

Pick the Best Time to Start Your Diet

That time is right now. But you may want to delay a diet if the start of it is going to coincide with a festive occasion.

It's not wise to start a new nutrition program if you are going through a series of emotional problems or dramatic upheavals in your life.

If your primary reason for following the Pain-Free Diet is weight loss, remind yourself that putting things off may mean extra ounces, or even pounds, to cope with later.

Think Thin and Pain-Free

Keep imagining a new, healthy, pain-free, and slimmer you. Build a mental picture of what you want yourself to feel and look like, and how much more you are going to enjoy life in the future.

Make Lists

Make a list of all the positive benefits you expect to receive from the Pain-Free Diet and how these benefits are going to affect your life. Draw up a list of things you expect to do that you weren't able to do before, especially in the fields of mobility, exercise, and possibly sports.

From the weight-loss point of view you might want to make a note of being less self-conscious, having more energy, and feeling healthier than you ever believed you could.

Exercise

Although you will learn many specific exercises in the next chapter that are designed especially for pain problems, you might want to consider joining an exercise or dance class as an additional motivation.

If your pain is too severe to allow this at the start of the diet, you might want to make a note of this as a future possibility as you reduce the level of your pain and your muscles and joints become more limber through our gentle exercises.

Buy Some Clothes in Smaller Sizes

This applies to dieters who also want to lose a fair amount of weight. You can achieve two aims here. First, buying the clothes you eventually want to fit into will act as a further incentive to maintain the diet program. Second, if you wear these clothes around the house and are aware of their tight fit (by checking a mirror periodically for bulges), this is a further weight-loss motivator.

New clothes can also act as a good monitor of how you are actually doing on the diet as you see the excess fat melting away.

Rewards

Every time you lose a pound or so, reward yourself. This can be as simple as a little gift or a special treat. Set yourself weight-loss goals in stages and reward yourself when you reach each one.

Another little trick is to promise yourself a nice vacation when you reach your ideal weight.

Reminder Pictures

Cut out from magazines photographs of models you admire and would like to look like. You can even paste up old photos of yourself next to them to remind you of what you used to look and feel like.

Make Little Signs to Remind You of Your Goals

The simpler these are the better, and you can stick them up around the home or workplace. They can be made out of colored sticky paper with little messages like "I Can Do It," "Think Pain-Free," "Slim Is In," or whatever triggers your motivation.

Junk the Junk Foods

Throw out all the snacks, junk foods, and any other food supplies that might prejudice your new diet plans. These will only act as temptation when you hit weak moments —and there will be some! If these tempters are not there, you'll be less likely to have them preying on your mind.

If you live in a household where other people find it impossible to live without junk food, think about putting these items in plain plastic, metal, or even paper containers that don't temptingly display their wares.

Begin to stock up on all the foods you are going to find beneficial to your new nutritional lifestyle. Make a big thing of this, like a specially planned trip to the grocery store, and consider it a turning point in your life.

Togetherness

Seek out a special friend, family member, or colleague who you know might also want to start on a new dietary regimen or weight-reduction program. This way there can be moral support for you both—even if it has to be over the telephone.

Don't Reveal Your Diet Plans Before You Start

Give it a good chance to show results. It's not a sound idea to inform friends and relatives outside the immediate home environment that you're going on a diet plan. Avoid the chance of negative feelings or comments. This may sound contrary to the last piece of advice, but the fewer people who know about your diet plans, the fewer people you may find dissuading you.

You'll gain instant support when friends see how good you are beginning to look and feel after you've been on the diet for a week or so.

Now that you've discovered some easy ways to springboard yourself into the diet, we'll look at more ideas to help you stick successfully to the diet, with a little help from yourself and your friends.

HINTS FOR STAYING WITH IT

Having support is one of the most constructive ways of sticking to a diet plan. In the following suggestions you'll find many that incorporate the help of family or friends once the ball is rolling.

- Keep away from the bathroom scales. Weight does fluctuate from day to day, so if losing weight is your prime goal it can be a negative experience to compare your weight every day. The best advice is to use the scales once every ten days or so; then you will certainly see positive and optimistic results.
- Increase your activity. This in itself helps the body burn

off excess weight and get back into shape, even if it's only a fifteen-minute walk every day.

- If you get tempted to break the diet, sit down with a friend or spouse and draw up a list of pros and cons for continuing the diet. You'll be surprised how the pros outweigh the cons.
- Persuade your family and friends not to eat any tempting and fattening foods in your presence.
- Try not to talk about the diet with friends—especially those who have tried other diets and failed—unless it's in positive terms. You may not have too much to report at the start, and this is a critical time during which friends may side with you if you are the least bit negative. Wait until you really start feeling and showing the results. Never reveal how much weight you've lost until you reach your ideal weight.
- Instead of going out for a snack or drink with a spouse or friend, try another activity, like taking in a movie, going for a walk, or even browsing at the library.
- If you happen to walk to work passing a bakery, deli, or any other food store that might offer tempting smells or sights, change your route.
- If you happen to work around food, arm yourself each day with nutritional lo-cal snacks that fit into the diet. Vegetable and fruit snacks are a good idea in helping to avoid the problem foods around you.
- Purposely plan your shopping and your menus to specific amounts of food so you don't keep stocking the refrigerator with tempting leftovers.
- Try to keep out of the kitchen as much as possible. If you have a spouse who's a whiz in the kitchen, let that person prepare all the meals, including yours.
- Remove from view around the home all food magazines or glossy magazines that carry tantalizing full-color food ads. One look at an ad displaying a mouth-watering chocolate cake can cause an endless craving that could detract from your diet.

- Encourage yourself to accept dinner and party invitations. Just because there's lots of food and drink around doesn't mean you have to participate as fully as everybody else. The best idea is to have a nutritious snack before you attend, as this will dull your appetite and prevent overeating.

- Try to avoid ethnic restaurants where, besides the dishes being full of rich sauces and gravies, it's very difficult to get an accurate calorie, protein, carbohydrate, and fat count on the foods you eat. Stick to restaurants where you'll find the nutritional mathematics easier to handle.

- When dining out, always remember to take along your tryptophan and vitamin supplements. These will not perform their function effectively if they are ingested long after the meal.

- Do not skip breakfast or lunch. Both of these meals are equally important to the success of the Pain-Free Diet. You may be avoiding a few calories, but it's going to undermine your pain-free potential.

- A spouse or a friend should be supportive, but if you are out socially they should avoid telling anyone that you are on a diet. This just leads to "friends" being inquisitive and trying to embarrass you into eating something you don't need. The stock reply should be simply "I'm just not hungry right now."

- Utilize a little handwritten sign stuck to the refrigerator door telling you what nutritious snacks are available inside and reminding you what not to touch.

These are just a few little tricks you can use. You will probably be able to think up many more yourself.

12
PAIN-FREE EXERCISES

We've already explained why pain-free exercises should go hand in hand with the Pain-Free Diet, but there's also another point you should be aware of to help reinforce your exercise motivation: Pain tolerance goes up with regular exercise, and this further enhances your pain-free potential.

Most people believe exercise has to hurt to help. But there are several ways a person can maintain good health and fitness that are as natural to the body as eating and sleeping.

It's particularly important for chronic-pain sufferers to keep limber and reduce tension—an integral part of pain— as well as develop a winning attitude to defeat the pain in their lives.

We have developed the Six-Point Exercise Plan for Living without Pain. All of the simple, gentle exercises take only minutes a day, and can be done safely by anyone.

Beginning with deep-breathing exercises, you will learn how to regulate your breathing to diffuse daily stress and gradually increase your body's strength, energy, and endurance.

The limbering-up exercises will give you a good basic program for exercising your joints, starting with the head and neck, continuing through the upper torso, arms, and hands, down to the legs and feet.

Many of these exercises were developed by the National Arthritis Foundation for sufferers of rheumatoid arthritis and osteoarthritis. And arthritis sufferers in particular should try to do them daily because joints that aren't used tend to stiffen up and cause pain.

In the section on painkillers you will learn how to adjust your lifestyle and prevent pain before it starts, including ways to make walking more comfortable, methods for reducing the stress of long-distance travel, and tricks to take best advantage of your limited strength and energy.

We've also included a section with mental exercises that you may find particularly beneficial for reducing tension and the inevitable pain that goes along with it. It's really mind over matter, but for many this is just the medicine.

One of the hottest developments in pain relief today is as old as civilization itself—water. Water straight from the tap is being used to relieve the aches and pains of millions suffering from swollen joints, torn ligaments, back injuries, sprains and strains, cancer, and even cold sores. This section will explain how many of you can get rid of your aches and pains with the turn of a faucet.

Since no exercise program can work properly without a change in attitude, the final section will give you a few simple rules to develop a better health outlook. Remember, no program, no matter how good, will work unless you fit it into your lifestyle. So read through the exercises, tips, and suggestions, and then adapt the parts of the exercise plan to suit your own personal needs.

In just a matter of days you will be amazed at how good you feel!

THE 6-POINT PLAN FOR LIVING WITHOUT PAIN

1. Breathing—the Antistress Link to Your Heart

Most people tend to think of stress in terms of major life catastrophes, like death, loss of a job, serious illness, and divorce. But it's the little stresses we cope with every day, like being late for work, overcooking dinner, or waiting in those inevitably long lines at the bank or supermarket, that eventually add up to killer proportions.

Research indicates that on the average a person reacts to stress between 125 and 150 times a day. And every time this happens, the body responds by sending a surge of adrenaline through its channels.

If this buildup isn't released in some way, it eventually snowballs. When you consider that this goes on in the body seven days a week, fifty-two weeks a year, it's no wonder stress is one of our biggest unseen killers and sources of pain.

While the responses themselves are natural, it's their effect on the weakest body links that create the problem. An individual with a bad heart, for example, could develop serious cardiovascular problems. Another may suffer from excruciating tension headaches. And still another could be prone to gastrointestinal problems.

Fortunately, you can help prevent tension buildup by breathing it away. Efficient breathing is an important link between the level of your blood pressure and your heart. When you get nervous or upset, your breathing tends to speed up and become irregular, triggering the body's stress reaction. But by teaching yourself to breathe deeply, you can force your respiration back to normal.

If you practice the following stress-reduction exercises

every day, stress will have less chance to accumulate in your body.

However, for the exercises to be most effective, don't wait until the end of the day when you may have built up so much tension that it's almost impossible to diffuse it. Instead, try to do them every hour or immediately at the onset of a particularly stressful situation.

All of the following exercises can be effective in reducing stress and producing a feeling of well-being. It's just a matter of finding the one that works best for you.

- Inhale deeply through both nostrils while keeping your mouth closed. Hold to the count of four. Then exhale slowly. Repeat three times.
- While keeping your eyes closed, inhale to the count of four. Then exhale slowly, thinking about the way the air feels as you slowly breathe in and out. Repeat three times.
- Close your eyes once again and inhale deeply, taking three or four short breaths. Then exhale quickly through your mouth. Repeat three times.
- While holding a finger over one nostril, breathe as deeply as you can through the other. Hold to the count of four. Then exhale slowly. Repeat with the other nostril.
- Hold the palm of your hand vertically in front of your mouth. Then inhale deeply and exhale slowly while concentrating on the warm air hitting your palm. Repeat five times.

2. Limbering Up

The following easy-to-do exercises recommended by the National Arthritis Foundation can help you move and feel better. Once your body is physically fit, you'll automatically be able to adopt a healthier mental attitude toward your specific health problem.

Since there is no special clothing or equipment required, you can begin whenever you're ready.

HEAD AND NECK

- Sit or stand in a comfortable position. Slowly rotate your head first to one side and then to the other, as far as you can reach. Do this twice a day.
- While keeping your eyes tightly closed, clench your jaws and make a face. Hold this position for four seconds. Then let go—all at once. Repeat four times. (This exercise is particularly good for those individuals suffering from headaches.)

NECK AND SHOULDERS

- Slowly raise your shoulders up and hold for two to three seconds. Then release. Repeat six times.
- Clasp your hands behind your head and move your head slowly from side to side. Repeat six times.

UPPER TORSO

- While standing up straight, clasp your hands behind your head. Then slowly stretch upward as if you're trying to reach the ceiling. Repeat six times. (This exercise is especially good for loosening up stiff joints.)
- While sitting in front of a table or desk, push away from it using your arms and hands. Then slowly lower your head to your chest and breathe deeply. Repeat six times.

BACK

- Lie flat on the floor, with your hands at your sides. Slowly raise your right leg as far as you can reach without bending your knee. Then lower. Repeat with your left leg. Try starting with three repetitions per leg and gradually increase your limit to ten. (This exercise is particularly good for sufferers from low back pain.)

- While standing or sitting in a comfortable position, arch your back and slowly raise your right hand as far as it will go while dropping your head to the left. Relax. Repeat arching your back, this time raising your left hand as far as it will go, while dropping your head to the right. Repeat three times.

HANDS, FINGERS, AND ELBOWS

- While sitting at a table or desk that you can lean across, reach over and place your hands on the other side, palm down, so that your fingers are dangling over the edge. Now extend and flex your fingers ten times. Repeat ten times.
- In the same position, move your hands, palms down, to the edge of the desk or table so the second finger joints rest at the edge. Then slowly extend and flex one finger at a time until you've done all ten. Repeat ten times.
- Stand facing a wall and extend both arms forward at shoulder height, while placing both hands on the wall. Then move your body forward, bending at the elbows as far as you can go. If you can, try to touch your shoulders to the wall. Repeat six times.

WAIST

- While standing straight, place both hands on your hips and slowly rotate your body first to one side, then the other. Repeat six times.

LEGS AND FEET

- While sitting or standing in a comfortable position, curl and uncurl your toes while pretending that you're trying to pick up some imaginary marbles. Repeat ten times.

- While sitting in a comfortable position, extend your leg slowly until it is as straight as you can get it. Then return to the starting position. Repeat ten times.
- While sitting in a comfortable position, bring up your right leg, put both arms around the knee, and hug it as close to your chest as you can. Hold for four seconds. Relax. Repeat with left leg.

3. Commonsense "Painkillers" for the Less Mobile

If you are an arthritis victim or suffer from chronic pain due to back or bone and joint injuries, you can prevent a lot of needless discomfort simply by taking a preventive approach to your daily activities.

Following are some suggestions to get you thinking. You can probably come up with many more.

- Save pressure and stress on your legs and feet by applying for a handicapped parking sticker so you can park closer to buildings; ask to be seated closest to the front door in restaurants and movie theaters in order to save steps; when cleaning house, do one floor at a time—don't switch up and down floors; if you have trouble walking, ask your doctor for advice about using an ambulatory device; when walking, avoid unnecessary stress on your knees and hips by sticking to soft surfaces, *i.e.*, grassy areas, carpeting, etc.; and when shoe shopping, make sure to select shoes that fit by checking the support on your arches, the way the shoes cushion the balls and heels of your feet, and if the front soles are flexible enough to give for an easy push-off.
- Save stress on your hands, arms, and fingers by using timesaving electric gadgets in your kitchen; avoid ironing by buying wash-and-wear clothing and bedding; when opening a door, push it with your hip instead of your hand; when carrying a heavy object, try putting most

of the weight on your shoulder instead of your hands; don't buy medication with childproof caps; get a car-starting device for the handicapped that you can use to turn on your ignition.

- Save your energy by taking a short, twenty-minute nap every day; try resting your injured or inflamed joints as often as you can during the day; keep track of your activity levels and try to schedule your heaviest work loads at the time of day you feel best.

- Eliminate painful joints due to prolonged periods of traveling by shifting your position every half hour or more. If you can, get up, stretch, and walk around. Carry a small pillow and use it to prop up the small of your back against the seat. Then sit as far back in the seat as possible so that your joints will line up correctly and prevent stress and fatigue.

- Don't forget to try minimal exercises if you can. When a joint is not sufficiently used, it will become stiff and sore. Even if you can't do much, you can still find some moderate activities that could make all the difference between getting up in the morning feeling stiff and sore or raring to go. (See the previous section on limbering-up exercises.)

4. Mental Exercises

The following five mental imagery exercises are often found by many people to be relaxing and to ease tension and stress.

1. Close your eyes and imagine your shoes are glued to the floor . . . so stuck that you can't move or lift them. Concentrate on this as long as you comfortably can. (This exercise is very effective in lowering heart rate.)

2. Close your eyes and imagine a favorite place you'd like to be . . . the beach, the mountains, etc. Then just let your mind wander while you fantasize about the scen-

ery. Concentrate on this as long as you can. (This exercise is very effective in lowering blood pressure.)

3. Close your eyes and imagine that your muscles have gone slack, leaving your body as floppy as a rag doll. Let yourself completely relax and think about this feeling for as long as you comfortably can.

4. Close your eyes tight and tense your body. Starting with your toes, your thighs, your stomach, your buttocks. Pull them all in. Hold for four seconds and then let go. Repeat six times.

5. Close your eyes and talk to your body. Say, "I am going to relax the muscles in my face. My shoulders are beginning to feel limp," etc. Continue doing this until you have "talked" to each part of your body.

5. Water—Hot and Cold Relief

Everybody knows about the soothing comfort of a warm, relaxing bath or the exhilarating feeling of a cool sponge-down after a rigorous workout.

But when used together in a certain way, hot and cold water can become a temperature-control technique that's so effective that it can bring relief from several types of acute injuries faster than any other known medical tool.

Thermal therapy has been the mainstay of orthopedic physicians for treating professional athletes for years. Now research is showing that it can be equally effective as an adjunct for treating arthritis and headaches; and it can even hasten the healing of many types of injuries. In its most elaborate form (called whole body aqua-thermia), medical researchers are beginning to report favorable results in treating cancer patients.

But its most interesting applications seem to be in the

everyday aches and pains that any sufferer can treat in the privacy of his or her own home.

The hot/cold treatment works by increasing and decreasing the blood flow. For example, a person with an acute back sprain would first apply an ice pack to decrease the swelling, followed by heat to promote healing.

The process would take continued applications of ice, twenty minutes on and twenty minutes off until the swelling had gone down (usually within forty-eight hours). Then the heat packs would be applied in the same way. While heat treatments have been the mainstay for treating rheumatoid arthritis patients, the response was pretty iffy until the method was reversed.

Then, in a dramatic example of blessed relief, arthritic patients who were given cold treatments for four weeks in a controlled medical setting were able to move about more freely. Their range of pain-free motion increased from thirty to ninety degrees, and many were even able to throw away their painkillers.

What was this awesome technique? Nothing more than four ice cubes in a plastic bag filled with a quart of water and draped over the affected knee. (Although only one knee was treated at a time, patients reported relief in both.)

Similarly, research with headache sufferers has shown that relief could be just a cold shower away. By taking a hot shower followed by a cold shower at the onset of a headache, patients being treated at a California medical facility were able to beat their migraine blues. According to the researchers, this happens because cold water shrinks the swollen blood vessels in the head and interrupts the headache.

While cold is usually the first line of treatment recommended for bruises, sprains, strains, and swellings, followed by heat, a lot of the effectiveness of hot/cold therapy depends on timing (everybody knows about the importance of plunging a burned or bashed finger under cold water as soon as possible) and individual results (not every arthritic patient responds well to heat treatments).

It's a good idea to be flexible according to the recommendations of the National Arthritis Foundation. Application of heat has long been a recognized means of relief. But if you're not getting it, you may want to try cold.

Because of the growing interest in this area and the promising research, it's certainly worth turning on the tap the next time you want to get rid of your aches and pains.

6. Attitudes for a Pain-Free Outlook*

Many people who are overweight and suffer from chronic pain tend to be very sedentary. But if you develop a healthy attitude, you'll be surprised at how much you can accomplish. The following suggestions should get you going. The rest is up to you.

Be an Energy Burner. Whatever you do, try to do it with the most energy you can muster. When you set the table, walk around it, don't just lean over. The same goes for making the bed. If you have the choice between the stairs and the elevator, take the stairs. These little extras can burn up ten additional calories each time you do them. And if you do enough of them, you could use up as much as 100 calories a day. Over a year's time you could wind up ten pounds thinner simply because you were willing to work a little harder.

Avoid Shortcuts. When the phone rings, don't grab for the most convenient extension. Instead, walk to the next room. The caller will keep trying for a few extra rings. Park your car away from the door at work so you'll have to walk a few more yards. Give your dog one bonus walk each day. Pack away your food processor and chop those vegetables

---

Do not confuse these tips with those on page 206 for Commonsense Painkillers for the Less Mobile.

by hand. Get your lawn mower back from your neighbor and do the lawn yourself. Wash your car instead of having it done at a car-wash service. These are just a few suggestions (you can certainly think up hundreds more) to exercise your body without having to work hard at it.

Pretend You're an Athlete. Take out a subscription to a sports magazine you happen to like. Even though you may not be able to participate physically, the mental fantasy will keep you motivated to do whatever you can to keep in shape. You may also want to buy a couple of jogging outfits or workout sweats and wear them around the house. Once again, imagery can work wonders for your motivation.

Find Your Optimum Exercise Time. If you are in pain in the morning or before bedtime, don't pick either as your time to exercise because you'll never go back. Instead, find your best time of day. It may be after breakfast or right before dinner. Then when you feel at your best, push yourself to do a little extra.

Good Health Is the Most Important Priority. When in a restaurant or having dinner at a friend's home, don't be embarrassed to ask for specific foods or beverages prepared the way your diet requires.

The same applies to your exercise regimen. If you want to limber up at your desk in the office, don't feel awkward because everybody is watching you. The better you look and feel, the more likely they will want to join in.

13

SLEEP, DEPRESSION, AND MOOD

By now you know quite a lot about tryptophan and its crucial function in the production of serotonin, the key to our pain management.

As you are aware, tryptophan plays other important roles in the human theater of our everyday lives, including sleep, energy, mood, and depression. What follows is a look at some of the most recent research by other scientists probing the beneficial effects of manipulating the levels of tryptophan in the diet.

Another MIT pioneer of the amazing capabilities of tryptophan, Dr. John D. Fernstrom of the Laboratory of Brain and Metabolism, department of nutrition and food science, hints that human studies of tryptophan may only be scratching the surface of the amino acid's beneficial potential.

He points out, "For example, the administration of tryptophan to animals, either by injection or addition of the amino acid to the food supply, reportedly improves sleep, reduces locomotor activity, suppresses male homosexual behavior, and causes long-term reduction in dietary protein intake. Tryptophan administration also reduces blood pressure in hypertensive rats.

"In humans, tryptophan may act as a hypnotic and an antidepressant. Tryptophan also has a modest stimulatory effect on growth hormone secretion in humans."

SLEEP

The effects of tryptophan on sleep in man have been studied numerous times, and the overall opinion is that tryptophan is a potent regulator of sleep and is especially useful in the treatment of sleep disorders.

For years scientists and chemists have been searching for the ideal, side-effect-free sleeping potion, unfortunately without too much success.

Statistics released by the Department of Health and Human Services show that in 1978 twice as many deaths were caused by sleeping pills as by heroin.

"We are dealing with a serious and major health issue," stated Surgeon General Julius B. Richmond. "Figures reveal that twenty-four million Americans use prescription drugs or over-the-counter sleep remedies, and we must aim at prevention—stopping the unwise use of money and the unnecessary deaths that result."

Yes, sleeping potions can be deadly when abused, or misused accidentally, but their everyday dangers go much deeper. Commercially available sleeping pills—mostly narcotics—and over-the-counter preparations work as sleep inducers in varying degrees, but in a very undesirable way: They literally knock you out.

Why is this undesirable? You're getting your sleep, aren't you? The answer is yes, if you consider something akin to being in a coma sleep.

During sleep-time a very delicate and fascinating web of intricate activity takes place inside your brain. The body can recharge itself during a state of rest, but the brain needs to have sleep. The quality of this sleep is of prime importance to our mental well-being. The honest truth is that while sleeping pills do make you sleep, they often don't allow for the quality of sleep because of the very action they take. They can zonk out your brain completely, and it won't be able to perform the necessary recharging it does during natural sleep. You've effectively "pulled the plug" on the brain.

Some sleep experts like to compare the brain to a computer that is constantly "on-line," receiving millions—maybe billions—of pieces of new information each day. If it keeps accepting information at this rate without being able to catalog and file it, the whole system will eventually disintegrate into total chaos. So, the computer has to come "off-line" and go into what computer programmers like to call "housekeeping" mode. This is the time when no external messages are coming in and the computer can attend to the storing and filing in its memory banks.

It is believed that the brain works in a very similar way. To prevent an overload of unfiled information it must come off-line, and this happens during sleep. Now the brain can do its housekeeping without your ever realizing it. But with potent narcotic sleep inducers, it's almost the same as pulling the plug on the computer and shutting it down completely. That is why the quality of natural sleep is far superior to that produced by so-called sleep aids.

There is also strong support that the brain's housekeeping takes place during REM (rapid eye movement) sleep—the periods during sleep when we are actively dreaming. We all dream, often many distinctly separate dreams, each night. These dreams may not be entirely comprehensible if you are able to recall them once you are awake, but it appears that the visions drifting through your nighttime subconscious are all part and parcel of the brain's unique ability to tidy up the day's happenings while you are fast asleep.

Many experiments have been done to probe the effects of sleep deprivation, and examples abound of what happens when the brain suffers from lack of sleep and becomes over-loaded. Not only do we become irritable and confused, but irrationality, exhaustion, and extreme depression set in. Af-ter a few days without sleep people begin to hallucinate, and if sleep is not forthcoming they will show all the signs of, quite literally, going crazy.

It's easy to speculate that the hallucinatory part of sleep deprivation is the brain's way of forcing dreams through to the conscious mind in an effort to instigate the housekeep-ing process and to warn that if it doesn't get some time out pretty soon, something much more drastic will take place.

Because drug-induced sleep does not provide the quality sleep we need, many people with a sleeping-pill dependency report that they still feel tired and irritable in the daytime even though they've had a full night's sleep. Anybody that has overimbibed and fallen into an alcohol-precipitated sleep will probably tell you they were not able to recall having dreamed at all that night, and they most probably didn't. They'll also report that even though they may have had six or eight hours sleep the night before they feel as if they haven't slept a wink. They might also suffer from terrible mental depression. Of course, the aftereffects of alcohol on the body itself—especially the liver—don't help, but the result of the alcohol's effect on the brain can be even more severe. Keep doing that every day and anybody, no matter who he is, is going to face severe emotional problems sooner or later.

It's easy to see why sleep and its quality are extremely important to our mental well-being, and why problem sleep-ers need help that will induce natural slumber and not knockout sleep.

The Tryptophan Lullaby

The problem suffered by most insomniacs, from mild to severe, is the inability to fall asleep, or what is referred to as sleep latency. For any person who has to adhere to a rigid work schedule and be up at a specific time every morning, this disorder can create a living nightmare. And, of course, the more people worry about it, the worse their sleep latency problem becomes.

There are cures without having to resort to knockout pills. For some it is simply a matter of resetting their personal biological sleep clock and gradually advancing their bedtime around the twenty-four-hour clock until they reach a happy medium that suits their personal needs.

Then there's the old-fashioned way, the late-night glass of warm milk. It doesn't work! According to MIT's Dr. Richard Wurtman, it's just a myth. And the reason—as we recognize from our understanding of tryptophan's competition with other amino acids—is simplicity itself. Milk is rich in the proteins that contain both tryptophan and the other amino acids. Our natural sleep inducer (tryptophan) is still fighting for space to get across the blood-brain barrier because milk contains high numbers of those competing amino acids.

The ideal bedtime sleep enhancer, says Dr. Wurtman, is tryptophan together with a high-carbohydrate snack to create a helpful insulin level, which assists tryptophan's passage against the competition.

Recorded Clinical Effects on Mild Adult Insomnia

One of the most interesting series of studies of the effects of tryptophan on sleep latency has been conducted by Dr. Ernest Hartmann, M.D., at the famed Sleep and Dream Laboratory at Boston State Hospital in Massachusetts. Together with Dr. Cheryl Spinweber, Dr. Hartmann treated a number of patients with sleep onset problems by giving them supplements of tryptophan just before bedtime. The result: They went to sleep faster and slept better.

Reported Dr. Hartmann, "What emerged from these studies was that L-tryptophan reduces sleep latency even at a dose of 1 gram at bedtime, at least in subjects who normally report a long sleep latency."

In one of Dr. Hartmann's studies, fifteen normal male subjects, ages twenty-one to thirty-five, who reported sleep latencies of over thirty minutes were recruited for the study.

The subjects were to sleep individually in the laboratory all night for seven nights during which time polygraphic recordings charted exactly their time of sleep onset and the depths of sleep experienced during the night.

The first two experimental nights were considered adaptation nights. On the next five nights the subjects were given one of the following, twenty minutes before bedtime, assigned in a counterbalanced order: a placebo (twice), 250 mg of tryptophan, 500 mg of tryptophan, and 1 gm of tryptophan.

After the experiment was over all the subjects' sleep readings were analyzed. Dr. Hartmann found that when the 1 gm bedtime dose of tryptophan was administered, the "insomniacs," who previously had experienced trouble falling asleep in under thirty minutes, were nodding off on average in as little as fifteen to eighteen minutes.

"Clinically, it appears from this study and previous work that 1 gm of L-tryptophan is a dose that can be reliably counted on to reduce sleep latency in long latency subjects, and our clinical experience suggests that such a dose is indeed useful for mild short-term insomnia," reported Dr. Hartmann.

... And Babies Too

New findings recently published by Boston physicians Dr. Michael Yogman and Dr. Steven Zeisal in the *New England Journal of Medicine* indicate that tryptophan can work as well for sleeping babies as it does for adults. The physicians fed twenty healthy newborns with two different glucose solutions and the commercial feeding formula Similac.

The first glucose solution contained tryptophan. The second was laced with the amino acid valine (one of the neutral amino acids that competes with tryptophan to get to the brain).

Drs. Yogman and Zeisal then compared the babies' sleep patterns and found that those who had been administered the glucose-tryptophan solution entered the first stage of sleep on average fourteen minutes sooner than those who drank Similac. They then went on to enter the second stage of sleep twenty minutes sooner. But the infants who had the valine-glucose solution entered these sleep stages significantly later than did the Similac babies.

The reason the valine babies didn't fare too well in these slumber stakes, concluded the physicians, was that the natural antagonistic action of valine to tryptophan interfered with the absorption of plasma tryptophan from the blood and therefore decreased serotonin levels in the brain.

Although Similac also contains tryptophan, the doctors believe the unique combination of glucose (a carbohydrate) maximized the efficiency of tryptophan, allowing more of it to enter the brain to boost serotonin production.

Severe Insomniacs

In a review of current research that has employed tryptophan-boosting to help chronic insomniacs, Dr. Cheryl Spinweber and Dr. Dietrich Schneider-Helmert of the Naval Health Research Center in San Diego, California, report promising results for tryptophan as a natural treatment for insomnia.

In several studies where tryptophan was administered in ranges of 1 gram to 7.5 grams to severe insomniacs shortly before their bedtimes, beneficial effects were continually recorded.

Commented Dr. Spinweber, "These sleep laboratory studies have confirmed the efficacy of L-tryptophan in chronic insomniacs . . . a therapeutic effect has been demonstrated (in younger sleep onset insomniacs) with a single administration of L-tryptophan at doses as low as 1 gram. Severe chronic insomniacs, on the other hand, seem to require repeated administration until sleep improvement occurs."

Dr. Spinweber made the following positive notes about tryptophan's role in sleep in her report.

- The lowest effective dose of L-tryptophan in acute treatment is one gram. It appears that the minimum effective dose may vary depending on the severity of the insomnia. To obtain reliable effects on sleep latency in acute treatment L-tryptophan should be administered at least thirty to forty-five minutes before bedtime at a dose between one gram and five grams, depending on the degree of sleep disturbance.
- Chronic insomniacs appear to respond to low doses of L-tryptophan only after repeated administration. Perhaps the disturbed regulatory system of the chronic insomniac is too rigid to react immediately to a therapeutic increase of a natural agent.
- The lack of side effects, even with high doses, in administration over long periods of time, or in especially sensitive populations, is of great practical value.
- There are no indications of the development of tolerance under continuous long-term administration of L-tryptophan.
- In the range of therapeutic doses, L-tryptophan does not affect the normal distribution of sleep stages.

It seems apparent from the growing wealth of research on sleep and tryptophan that it can be a potent enhancer of sleep, even at very small doses, in a normal, or mildly disturbed, sleep population. In other words, we believe, those occasional restless nights can be eliminated with the Pain-Free Diet program.

Chronic severe insomniacs may find that the calming-sleep effectiveness of the Pain-Free Diet takes a few days from its start to become fully effective. If you are suffering from severe or chronic sleep disturbance the message here is to give the Pain-Free Diet a little time for the body to begin its changes and reap the natural benefits. Don't give up if it doesn't work for the first couple of nights; your body has to correct imbalances that may have existed for years.

DEPRESSION—WHAT IS IT?

Depression is recognized by the medical profession as falling into two distinct forms: as a normal mood, and as a serious mental disorder.

Everyone experiences transient depression. It's a mood change, and it's natural. Some states of depression quite normally follow an exciting or pleasurable experience, especially if it has been long awaited and anticipated—maybe the homecoming of a loved one, a special party event or gift, or a well-deserved vacation. But you soon snap out of this malaise, which is usually short-lived, as other interesting or exciting events come along in your life. This type of depression may well serve a distinct purpose; you have to experience the lows to appreciate the highs.

If you were running around every day in a constant state of euphoria, chances are that eventually even this pleasing experience would start to look commonplace, and you'd be on a never-ending upward search for some unattainable emotional Holy Grail, like a drug addict.

Obviously, there have to be an emotional safeguard and a lull in our emotional levels. A minor depression seems to serve this purpose.

But some people suffer from more protracted periods of depression without it falling into the category of a serious mental illness. It is now becoming apparent from recent research that the reduced levels of important neurotransmitters, especially serotonin, may be the cause of unnecessary long periods of depression.

There's also an undeniable link between sleep and depression, and between pain and depression. What makes this such a fascinating avenue of research is that they are all influenced by the levels of brain serotonin.

Because pain is so often associated with depression, and depression with pain, the Pain-Free Diet can kill two unwanted conditions with one stone. We'll analyze this a little later in the chapter, but first it's important to understand the differences between depressions because we do not intend to suggest, or do we believe, that the Pain-Free Diet is an acceptable treatment for a depression that has its roots in a serious mental disorder. We stress that if you feel your depression may be of this type, it's essential you seek professional help.

How to Recognize It

There's no doubt you'll recognize normal depression: It's a humdrum world; you feel in the doldrums; there doesn't seem to be anything to look forward to; little things niggle you; you feel tired and listless; you might have trouble sleeping; you're bored; and you might be restless. You're depressed.

Dr. Philip A. Berger, assistant professor in the department of psychiatry and behavioral sciences at Stanford University School of Medicine, gives the following elegant description of depression: "The term depression is used to describe both a normal mood and a serious mental disorder. As a normal mood, depression refers to the transitory feelings of sadness, grief, disappointment, loneliness, or discouragement that everyone feels during the difficult times of life.

"As a mental disorder, depression is an illness with many symptoms, only one of which is sadness. Those with depression have changes in moods, thinking patterns, motor activity, and behavior. They also have somatic or physical symptoms and frequently have suicidal ideas that can tend to self-destructive behavior.

"The mood in depressed individuals (as a mental illness) is variable but includes profound sadness and often a loss of ability to feel pleasure. The ideas, activities, and relationships that usually bring pleasure can seem empty and hollow. The changes in thinking patterns lead to pessimism about the future and low self-esteem. Depressed people often deny their accomplishments or feel unworthy of current achievements.

"Feelings of low self-esteem or worthlessness combine with pessimism to rob them of their motivation, making it difficult to maintain either their jobs or interpersonal relationships."

Dr. Berger also points out that physical symptoms often accompany severe depression, including sleep anomalies and pains: "Physical symptoms are often a prominent part of the depression syndrome. Those with severe depression often have no appetite and lose weight.

"Sleep disturbance is another common symptom, causing insomnia, restless nights, and early morning awakening. In severe depression a patient often wakes at 3 or 4 A.M. and is unable to get back to sleep.

"Some depressed patients also experience constipation, dry mouth, tight feelings in the chest, and aches and pains, particularly headaches and backaches. Many depressed people lose interest in sexual activity, and depressed women often have changes in their menstrual cycle."

It is clear in some mildly depressed subjects that the pain or the sleeplessness may lead to the depression, rather than the other way around. The depression may, however, be the trigger for the pain and sleep disorders. The root of the whole syndrome could also be an initial depletion of brain serotonin caused by a tryptophan-poor diet, or a diet in which tryptophan is not able to achieve maximum potential. There are numerous other factors that can come into play, including other chemicals involved with neurotransmitters.

But the latest research into depression and serotonin levels in the brain shows some very intriguing results.

Autism, Down's Syndrome, Manic Depression

Researchers in the psychiatric field are also discovering exciting ramifications in the tryptophan-serotonin connection.

Previous studies by a number of scientists appeared to show a distinct link between a malfunction of the serotonin production chain and Down's syndrome. Other researchers noticed the same serotonin disruption traits in manic depressives.

Of course, the question has to be asked, "Could Down's syndrome be caused by the insufficient production of serotonin—or is the lack of serotonin a result of Down's syndrome?" We don't know the answers yet, but this very significant factor may well lead to a better understanding of the condition, and possibly a remedy.

A carefully detailed study conducted in Japan reveals that autistic children show a distinct abnormality in metabolism of serotonin in the brain—and the lower the mental development of the child, the greater the metabolic disruption seems to be.

At the Fukishima Medical College in Japan, Dr. Yoshiko Hoshino and colleagues studied thirty-seven autistic children and compared their blood tryptophan levels with sixty-seven normal children and adults. What they discovered and published in 1984 could possibly be the start of a major breakthrough, certainly in the understanding of autism. The study showed that autistic children displayed much higher amounts of plasma-free tryptophan in their bloodstreams. This startling discovery led the researchers to the conclusion that something was going wrong with the metabolism of tryptophan and that the increased levels were possibly present because tryptophan was not being converted through the natural process into the all-important neurotransmitter serotonin.

Obviously, there had to be a breakdown somewhere in the tryptophan system, and the necessary levels of serotonin vital to the brain's correct functioning were not being manufactured. Exactly where this breakdown is occurring has yet to be pinpointed.

Dr. Hoshino confirms, "Our present study shows that the plasma concentration of free TRP (tryptophan) was significantly higher in autistic children than in normal children or adults . . . the lower the mental development of autistic children, the higher the plasma-free TRP level tended to be."

The scientist adds, "The supposition of defective serotonin synthesis, particularly from 5-HTP to serotonin, appears to be cogent in explaining the elevated plasma-free TRP level in autistic children."

Much further research has to be conducted to understand exactly what part the tryptophan-serotonin mechanism plays in autism, but this significant research certainly appears to hold out potential new hope for parents of autistic children.

TRYPTOPHAN AND SEROTONIN: THE LONG-TERM VIEW

Serotonin acts like a natural hypnotic agent in sleep, its important role in depression is now being recognized, and we know its key role in pain control and other vitally important areas of our lives. What are the long-term prospects of tryptophan therapy?

Sleep scientist Dr. Hartmann, who is also professor of psychiatry at Tufts University School of Medicine, is enthusiastic about the long-term effects of treating depressed patients with serotonin-boosting levels of tryptophan.

At the moment tryptophan is viewed by the FDA as a food supplement, and with that classification no medical claims can be made by manufacturers about its benefits.

This situation could soon change, however. As more scientists study tryptophan and its roles, and are able to offer valid clinical findings as to its importance to the human condition, the FDA may accept tryptophan as a therapeutic device. It would then have to fall into one of the many FDA drug classifications and could be prescribed by a physician for a specific medical condition or ailment.

Until this happens a physician can offer you guidance and suggestions on the benefits of tryptophan, and the Pain-Free Diet is available for you to take full advantage of it.

In some countries the story is different. One of these is Great Britain, where the benefits of tryptophan therapy have long been recognized and accepted by medical professionals.

It must be pointed out that short-term studies are one thing, and long-term studies with a large population are another. The fear of any medical professional is that a substance may prove to have side effects, be toxic, or become addictive in the long term. British studies help to subdue this fear.

Dr. Hartmann has ongoing personal communications with British physicians using tryptophan for the relief of depression and with the Medicines Council of Great Britain, which approves its administration. He reports, "L-tryptophan is already in use on a long-term basis as an antidepressant in Great Britain."

And Dr. Hartmann adds, "Doses of 6–9 grams a day have been taken for a period of many months by several thousand patients with reports of very few side effects, and no serious ones.

"No psychological symptoms have been reported during these periods by the normal subjects in our studies: no problems on withdrawal have been reported by sources in Great Britain. This would lead one to hope that addiction and withdrawal problems would be minimal or absent with L-tryptophan."

Studies at the Pain Unit of the Veterans Administration Hospital in San Diego, California, and the department of psychiatry at the University of California in San Diego have also investigated the double link of pain and depression, and tryptophan.

The subjects of these studies were men, ages twenty-two to sixty, who had been hospitalized at the Veterans Administration Hospital for a variety of pain-related problems, mostly musculoskeletal (disc disease), and all of long duration.

They were divided into three groups, one group that received either L-tryptophan or 5-HTP (5-hydroxytryptophan, the second stage of tryptophan conversion before it becomes serotonin). In this group the researchers were able to note an observable decrease in pain levels and reduced levels of depression after the administration of the serotonin precursors.

One of the researchers, Dr. Richard A. Sternbach, explained, "In man, chronic pain is often associated with depression. We hypothesize that a common mechanism to account for increasing pain and depression with chronicity may lie in depletion or decreased activity of brain 5-HT (serotonin)."

The serotonin study was performed to test this hypothesis. Dr. Sternbach adds, "The results suggest that increased brain serotonin activity causes decreased pain . . . and seems to do so by increasing pain tolerance."

Other scientists have noticed an interesting similarity between the way serotonin-boosting affects the mentally depressed and the way common antidepressant drugs act. These drug compounds, known as tricyclics, are the most commonly used medications prescribed for depression.

"Tricyclics take 2 to 4 weeks to alter the symptoms of severe depression, but they are effective in about 70 percent of patients," states depression expert Dr. Philip A. Berger. "In most cases tricyclics cause a complete remission of depressive symptoms: they improve mood, restore confidence, relieve the numerous physical symptoms, and eliminate suicidal thinking. Some patients may fail to respond to one tricyclic but will respond to another."

But why is this so important? Listen further to Dr. Berger.

"Despite an impressive quantity of data accumulated over the last twenty years, the exact mechanism of action of tricyclics is unknown. The most important hypothesis is that tricyclics increase the functional activity of the brain neurotransmitters norepinephrine and serotonin."

And he adds, "This hypothesis, which is supported by several pharmacological and physiological findings, states that depression is due to a functional underactivity or deficiency of these neurotransmitters."

It seems that the link between serotonin and pain, sleep, mood, and depression is indeed becoming clearer. With the help of the natural serotonin-boosting action of tryptophan, is there really any reason why anyone should continue to suffer from sleep problems, mild depression, and pain?

14

NEW HOPE FOR MIGRAINE AND CHRONIC-HEADACHE SUFFERERS

Because the number of sufferers from migraine and chronic headaches runs into the multimillions in this country, we feel that the latest exciting research into the role of tryptophan in migraine and headache relief deserves a chapter of its own.

The present studies are rather limited, but from all indications of the work already conducted by physicians in Finland and Italy the tryptophan-serotonin link may well offer new hope to sufferers of migraine and chronic headaches.

Over twenty million people are experiencing migraine attacks or chronic headaches this very day. You may be one of them. Although the exact chemical link between serotonin and migraine headaches has still to be fully understood, there is reason to hope that the boosting of brain serotonin can bring miraculous relief to sufferers—many of whom may have endured their affliction for years. The tryptophan-serotonin link with migraine and headache relief is one we should not ignore.

As you have already read in Chapter 3, ordinary foods can

be the cause of migraine attacks and headaches. You have seen that the actions of these foods as vasoconstrictors and vasodilators on the important blood vessels in the brain, head, neck, and shoulders can cause excruciating pain attacks.

If you are a migraine or headache sufferer who has not considered specific foods as a potential source of your migraine and not known of the elimination techniques recommended in Chapter 3, we strongly recommend you do so at this time. The Pain-Free Diet can help your problem, if not eliminate it altogether. But isn't it much more sensible to dispense with the offending foods first if they are the primary cause?

CLINICAL TESTS OF THE EFFECT OF TRYPTOPHAN

Many of the studies utilizing tryptophan- and serotonin-boosting have been conducted by scientists in Europe, where tryptophan is already recognized as a potent inhibitor of pain.

At Finland's University of Turka physicians have been probing the exciting effects tryptophan has on migraine sufferers, and they have come up with an extremely interesting reason as to why migraine victims suffer so much and for so long in individual attacks.

Dr. P. Kangasniemi and his colleagues in the university's department of neurology and clinical neurophysiology theorize that the onset of a migraine attack causes stress and this in turn releases albumin-bonded tryptophan already circulating in the blood, making more of it available for the brain to produce pain-modulating serotonin. But, as we have seen, sufficient amounts of free tryptophan supplies don't always exist in the bloodstream to produce enough serotonin to knock out the pain.

Explains Dr. Kangasniemi, "If there is not enough tryptophan available in blood circulation for brain serotonin turnover, and the protection against pain cannot be reached, then additional tryptophan may be necessary to prevent the migraine pain.

"Furthermore, if the brain serotonin turnover is already slow per se, the additional tryptophan should be even more necessary."

In a study of eight migraine patients, six female and two male, ages twenty-four to forty-nine, who had suffered from migraine for over ten years, all were given tryptophan and observed for three months. They were given a total of two grams of tryptophan each day in four doses of 500 mg.

At the end of the trial the scientists found that four of the eight patients who had suffered serious migraine symptoms reported significant relief after the administration of tryptophan, and continued to show additional improvements up to a year later during follow-up interviews. The other four migraine sufferers reported "feeling better" while on tryptophan, but the results were not as evident as with the sufferers of more severe pain. The doctors also reported no side effects during the study.

Dr. Kangasniemi states categorically, "Tryptophan seems to be a worthwhile alternative for a selective and still non-characterized group of migraine patients."

One of the foremost pioneer researchers of the migraine-serotonin link is Dr. Federigo Sicuteri of the University of Florence in Italy. Dr. Sicuteri and fellow researchers in the Headache Clinic of the department of clinical pharmacology report another fascinating finding: Available tryptophan in the blood shows an actual decrease during migraine attacks.

The importance of this finding is that it backs up the Finnish theory that tryptophan is indeed rushed to the brain during a migraine attack to bolster the serotonin level. The problem may be that severe migraine sufferers do not have sufficient amounts of tryptophan available in the blood to counteract the pain.

A conclusion that can be derived from this is that people may become severe migraine victims because they simply do not have adequate amounts of serotonin-boosting tryptophan. Conversely, it could be proposed that the person who suffers the occasional mild headache might but for the grace of adequate tryptophan supplies be a chronic-migraine sufferer.

There is also another thought-provoking finding by Dr. Sicuteri that might explain why migraine sufferers find very little relief from potent analgesic drugs, which would normally eliminate or reduce other forms of pain.

Explains Dr. Sicuteri, "It has been found in experimental animals that a deficiency of 5-hydroxytryptamine (serotonin) in the brain not only lowers the pain threshold but significantly reduces the analgesic activity of morphine."

This could mean that migraine sufferers face a double-edged sword: Not only do they have reduced levels of available tryptophan, but the drugs they take to counteract the pain also become virtually useless without the essential levels of serotonin and the sufficient supply of tryptophan to produce it.

The Italian scientists also discovered that some chemicals which can pass the blood-brain barrier act to lower the sensitivity to pain in sufferers of migraines—while these same chemicals do not have this effect in the population of non-migraine sufferers.

Two of these chemicals, reserpine and parachlorophenylalanine (PCPA), are known to lower the brain content of serotonin. When they are introduced into a normal population they have no effect on pain, but in the migraine sufferer they result in pain, and, in 20 percent of cases, pain in the limbs, trunk, shoulders, and neck, reports Dr. Sicuteri. In some cases the pains are extremely intense, but disappear when PCPA is discontinued, and reappear when it is administered once more.

We believe this is further evidence to show that migraine sufferers have an inherent susceptibility to a lack of brain serotonin, and this is made even more acute when serotonin antagonists are present in the bloodstream.

Obviously, this leads to a conclusion that among pain victims, migraine sufferers may find it most beneficial to boost serotonin levels through additional tryptophan and the optimum conditions offered to serotonin production by the Pain-Free Diet.

In Dr. Sicuteri's studies he and his colleagues have administered tryptophan in varying doses to more than 150 migraine and chronic-headache sufferers.

Here is a summary of their conclusions.

- Tryptophan administered intravenously in doses of 100 mg three times a day improves occasional headaches of the migraine type. Similar results were observed in oral doses of tryptophan of 1 to 3 grams.
- When tryptophan is administered by venous infusion in doses of 2 gm in 250 cc in two hours, pain was reduced, and dramatically so in 30 percent of intractable headaches.
- After the introduction of tryptophan therapy, sufferers who had developed resistance to powerful analgesics through long-term use, found the painkilling potency they had experienced previously, but lost, had returned.

These important new findings in the treatment and management of migraine and chronic headaches indicate that some migraine sufferers have a definite inadequacy of tryptophan and are more susceptible to foods or chemicals that can reduce brain serotonin. These substances quickly lose their effectiveness as analgesic painkillers to control migraine problems because of the lack of available brain tryptophan.

What's the answer? It's not going to do any harm to increase your daily supplies of tryptophan through the Pain-Free Diet, and for many migraine sufferers it could be the key to a new pain-free lifestyle that they never thought possible.

BIBLIOGRAPHY

Appenzeller, O. "Headache: clinical and pathogenic aspects." *Advances in Pain Research and Therapy*, 3 (1979) 345–58.

Baumann, P.; Schmocker, M.; Reyero, F.; Heimann, H. "Free and bound tryptophan in the blood of depressives." *Acta Vitaminologica Enzymologica* (Milano), 29 (1975) 255.

Berger, Philip A. "Medical treatment of mental illness." *Science*, 200 (1978) 974–81.

Bliznakov, Emile G. "Modification of the Immunological Responsiveness of Mice by Serotonin (5-hydroxy-tryptamine) and its Precursors." VII International Meeting of International Society for Neurochemistry. Abstracts, p. 239. Athens-Jerusalem, September 1979.

———. "Suppression of Friend Leukemia Virus Infection in Mice by Serotonin (5-hydroxy-tryptamine) and its Precursors." XII International Cancer Congress. Abstracts, Vol. 3, Workshop #63—Leukemia, p. 244. Buenos Aires, Argentina, October 1978.

Booij-Noord, H.; Orie, N. G. M.; Devries, K. "Serotonin (5-hydroxy-tryptamine) inhalation in patients with chronic, non-specific lung disease." *Scandinavian Journal of Respiratory Diseases*, 50 (1969) 301–308.

Crook, Joan; Rideout, Elizabeth; Browne, Gina. "The prevalence of pain complaints in a general population." *Pain*, 18 (1984) 299–314.

Fernstrom, J. D. "Effects of the diet on brain neurotransmitters." *Metabolism*, 26 (1977) 207–23.

233

————. "Neutral amino acids, neurotransmitters, and brain function. Human Nutrition Clinical and Biochemical Aspects." Proceedings of the 4th Arnold O. Beckman Conference in Clinical Chemistry (1981) 302–14.

————; Hammarstrom-Wilklund, B.; Rand, W. M.; Munro, H. N.; Davidson, C. S. "Diurnal variations in plasma concentrations of tryptophan, tyrosine, and other neutral amino acids: effect of dietary protein intake." American Journal of Clinical Nutrition, 32 (1979) 1912–22.

————, and Wurtman, R. J. "Brain serotonin content: increase following ingestion of carbohydrate diet." Science, 174 (1971) 1023–25.

Greenberg, Stanley, and Palmer, Gene C. "Biochemical basis of analgesia: metabolism, storage, regulation, and action." Dental Clinics of North America, 22 (1978) 31–46.

Growdon, John H.; Cohen, Edith L.; Wurtman, Richard J. "Treatment of brain disease with dietary precursors of neurotransmitters." Annals of Internal Medicine, 86 (1977) 337–39.

Hartmann, Ernest. "L-tryptophan: a rational hypnotic with clinical potential. American Journal of Psychiatry, 134 (1977) 366–70.

————, and Spinweber, Cheryl L. "Sleep induced by L-tryptophan: effect of dosages within the normal dietary intake." Journal of Nervous and Mental Disease, 167 (1979) 497–99.

Hoshino, Y.; Yamamoto, T.; Kaneko, M.; Tachibana, R.; Watanabe, M.; Ono, Y.; Kumashiro, H. "Blood serotonin and free tryptophan concentration in autistic children." Neuropsychobiology, 11 (1984) 22–27.

Kangasniemi, P.; Falck, B.; Langvik, Vivi-Ann; Hyyppa, M. T. "Levotryptophan treatment in migraine." Headache, 18 (1978) 161–66.

Meier, Albert H., and Wilson, John M. "Tryptophan feeding adversely influences pregnancy." Life Sciences, 32 (1982) 1193–96.

Salmon, S.; Fanciullacci, M.; Bonciani, M.; Sicuteri, F. "Plasma tryptophan in migraine." Headache, 17 (1978) 238–41.

Schneider-Helmert, D., and Spinweber, C. L. "Evaluation of l-tryptophan for treatment of insomnia: a review." Report No. 84-4. Naval Health Research Center, San Diego, California, 1984.

Seltzer, Samuel. "Foods, and food and drug combinations, responsible for head and neck pain." Cephalgia, 2 (1982) 111–24.

————; Dewart, Dorothy; Pollack, Robert L.; Jackson, Eric. "The effects of dietary tryptophan on chronic maxillofacial pain and experimental pain tolerance." Journal of Psychiatric Research, 17 (1983) 181–86.

————; Marcus, Richard; Stoch, Russell. "Perspectives in the control of chronic pain by nutritional manipulation." Pain, 11 (1981) 141–48.

————; Stoch, Russell; Marcus, Richard; Jackson, Eric. "Alteration of human pain thresholds by nutritional manipulation and l-tryptophan supplementation." Pain, 13 (1982) 385–93.

Sicuteri, Federigo. "Headache as the most common disease of the anti-nociceptive system: analogies with morphine abstinence." *Advances in Pain Research and Therapy*, 3 (1979) 359–65.

———. "Headache: disruption of pain modulation." *Advances in Pain Research and Therapy*, 1 (1976) 871–80.

Spinweber, C. L. "L-tryptophan in psychiatry and neurology." Report No. 80-3. Naval Health Research Center, San Diego, California, 1980.

Sternbach, Richard A.; Janowsky, David S.; Huey, Leighton Y.; Segal, David S. "Effects of altering brain serotonin activity on human chronic pain." *Advances in Pain Research and Therapy*, 1 (1976) 601–606.

Wurtman, J. J. *The Carbohydrate Craver's Diet*. Boston: Houghton Mifflin Company, 1984.

———, and Wurtman, R. J. "Suppression of carbohydrate consumption as snacks and at mealtime by difenfluramine or tryptophan." In *Anorectic Agents: Mechanisms of Actions, and of Tolerance*, ed. S. Garattini. New York: Raven Press, 1981.

Wurtman, Richard J. "Nutrients that modify brain function." *Scientific American*, April (1982) 50–59.

———. "The ultimate head waiter: how the brain controls diet." *Technology Review*, July (1984) 42–51.

———; Hefti, R.; Melamed, E. "Precursor control of neurotransmitter synthesis: clinical implications." *Pharmacological Review*, 32 (1981) 315–35.

INDEX

vitamins and minerals during, 116–117

Pain-Free exercises, 200–206
advantages of, 200–201
breathing, 202–203
limbering up, 203–206

Painkillers
appetite loss and, 182
nonmedical for less mobile, 206–207
reduction or elimination of, 2
spending on, 7
tryptophan supplementation and, 112
See also Over-the-counter medications

Pain medications. *See* Painkillers
Pain perception, and serotonin, 19
See also Pain threshold

Pain relief
carbohydrates and, 17, 50, 70
exercise and, 9–10
feverfew and, 27
nutrition and, 8
tryptophan and, 28
water therapy and, 201, 208–210

Pain threshold, 21–22
in clinical tests of tryptophan, 34
raising, 20–21
serotonin and, 19, 20–21
tryptophan and, 6

Pain tolerance
benefits of increasing, 22
essential foods and, 48
exercise and, 200
tryptophan and, 21, 32–34

Pantothenic acid, 58
Parachlorophenylalanine (PCPA), in migraine sufferers, 231
Paralysis, saxitoxin and, 42
Paraplegic pain, 11
Parkinson's disease, tryptophan and, 25–26
Partially complete proteins, 16–17, 49
Parties, eating at, 199
Phantom limb pain, 11
Phenylalanine, 29
Photographs, weight loss and, 195
Physical symptoms, of severe depression, 222

Physicians
Pain-Free Diet and, 3, 111–112
pain and visits to, 7

Pies. *See* Cakes, cookies, and pies exchange list

Polyunsaturated fatty acids, 18, 51
Postmenopausal women, depression and tryptophan metabolism in, 25
Pregnancy, tryptophan during, 23, 112–113
Premenstrual syndrome (PMS), tryptophan metabolism and, 25
Prescription drugs, problems with, 7
Proteins, 48–49
amino acids and, 15–16
brain tryptophan levels and, 29
calories and, 67–68
complete, 16
incomplete, 17
partially complete, 16–17
requirements, 49, 64–68, 104
and tryptophan, 212–213
See also Amino acids; Meats

Psychotics. *See* Mental illness
Pyridoxine, 57
and tryptophan supplementation, 101–102, 103–107

Rebound scurvy, 56
REM (rapid eye movement) sleep, 214
Reserpine, in migraine sufferers, 231
Restaurants, 199
Rewards, for weight loss, 195
Riboflavin, 56–57
Rice, flavor enhancers for, 181
Richmond, Julius B., 213

Salads, flavor enhancers for, 181
Salt, 59
Saturated fatty acids, 51
Saxitoxin, 42
Scales, use of, 197
Schizophrenics, blood levels of tryptophan in, 25
Schneider-Helmert, Dr. Dietrich, 218
Scurvy, 47
Seafood
and iodine, 60
saxitoxin in, 42
Seltzer, Dr. Samuel, 20, 32–34
Serotonin
asthma and, 113
and autism, Down's syndrome, and manic depression, 223–224
brain chemistry and, 24